Medical Cannabis Primer

For Healthcare Professionals

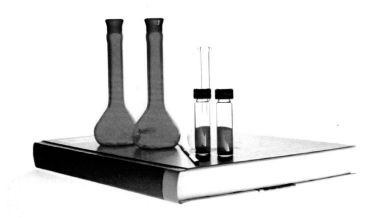

Laura Bultman, MD

and Kyle Kingsley, MD

Foreword

Background and Purpose

The book is intended as a brief guide to help health care providers understand the use of cannabis as medicine for patients with qualifying conditions. This volume is by no means comprehensive, but the goal is to give you the knowledge needed to assist your patients to find the best relief of their symptoms. It is apparent that a concise reference is needed by providers who need to provide sound advice to their patients, but have no experience to date with cannabis as medicine. In particular, we will focus on the research and evidence that exists for certain symptoms and conditions traditionally treated with cannabis derivatives and also the potential risks in the use of cannabis.

While politics and policy are mentioned this book, the focus is on providing simply the necessary medical knowledge to effectively use cannabis derivatives in the clinical setting. There is substantial evidence for the efficacy of cannabis in several conditions, but the presentation of that evidence is often colored by bias regarding cannabis in a political light.

From the Authors

Research on the subject of cannabis-based medicines both from the bench science and clinical therapeutic perspectives is compelling that this controversial field has tremendous value and an exciting future, and that medical science will continue striving toward defining it.

Like the authors, readers had no education about the endocannabinoid system or its manipulation in medical school, and likely had little education about pharmacognosy, the study of plants as medicine. With the development of medical cannabis programs in many states, it can be difficult to reconcile these new programs with long-held beliefs regarding avoidance of addictive drugs and the dangers of smoking.

How then do we approach these developments in cannabis medicine? Where can we find reliable information, untainted by political and other bias? Before recommending cannabis-based medicines to a patient, how is a provider to know the risks and benefits? Other clinicians have also likely found that it is difficult to separate the propaganda from the stigma from the science, and the information provided here is intended to bridge these informational gaps.

This book is certainly not intended to be static or all-inclusive, but aims to provide clinicians with the core knowledge necessary to discuss cannabis with patients and colleagues intelligently. Conducting a search for up-to-date, relevant medical works reveals that books written in the last five years are sparse, and are not often directed to a medical audience. This work represents a compilation of information from medical reference sources, bench science research, popular information and position statements, presented with the viewpoint of medical cannabis clinical professional.

Contents

Brief Medicinal Cannabis Lexicon

Budtender: the individual working the counter at medical marijuana dispensaries, who is employed to offer suggestions and advice to customers

Butane: as it applies to cannabis products, butane can be used to extract cannabinoids, terpenes and other lipophilic products from the whole cannabis plant. The residual butane solvent is then removed before consumption, resulting in an oily, sticky concentrate.

Cannabidiol (CBD): the second most well studied of the cannabinoids; it does not have psychotropic effects and has shown useful for a variety of inflammatory and neurologic disorders. As a constituent of cannabis species, it is most abundant in hemp varieties, but less common in cannabis strains that have been cultivated for higher THC and psychoactivity.

Cannabinoid: a family of terpenophenolic compounds unique to the cannabis plant. They can be further specified to be synthetic or of plant origin (phytocannabinoid). Mammals possess an endogenous system of ligands and receptors, termed the endocannabinoid system, upon which exogenous cannabinoids have a variety of effects. The naturally occurring or "raw" form of these cannabinoids exists with a carboxylic acid chain, which is most often removed with the application of heat to convert the raw form to the active form.

Decarboxylation: in reference to cannabis, this refers to the process required to convert the natural acidic form of cannabinoids to a physiologically active form by removing the carboxylic acid side chain. This does occur naturally with time, however the application of heat will greatly speed this process, and thus the most common routes of cannabis ingestion involve heat such as vaporizing, combustion or cooking.

Dispensary: a facility specializing in the distribution of either medicinal or recreational cannabis products. Unlike a pharmacy, they do not process true prescriptions for medical marijuana, but rather receive a medical recommendation for cannabis products in general. Personnel within the dispensary then make recommendations regarding the type of cannabis strain and delivery form, dose, and route of administration based on the needs of the patient.

Edibles: term for cannabis-containing products that are cooked or baked into more ordinarily edible forms, such as cookies or brownies.

Endocannabinoid: term for the widespread endogenous system of fatty-acid derived neuromodulators that affect intracellular signaling mainly in the nervous and immune systems. Receptors and intracellular proteins involved in natural endocannabinoid signaling are also sensitive to exogenous cannabinoids, which is the mechanism by which cannabis exerts its effects. Anandamide or *N*-arachidonoylethanolamine (AEA) and 2-arachidonoylglycerol (2-AG) are the two best known endocannabinoids, others include 2-arachidonylglyceryl ether (noladin ether), O-arachidonoyl-ethanolamine (virodhamine), and N-arachidonoyl-dopamine (NADA).

Ganja: Sanskrit for cannabis

Hash: traditionally this referred to a product made by collecting the resin glands of the cannabis plant, which have a concentrated amount of cannabinoids, and was more common practice in countries outside of the United States.

Hemp: term for Cannabis sativa varietals that lack THC, but retain other cannabinoids and can be grown for agricultural and medical use

Hybrid: as the term suggests, this refers to blending strains possessing different genetic characteristics into the final cannabis product in order to achieve desired effects

Indica: along with sativa, one of the main varieties of the *Cannabaceae* species. More often from a tropical source, the variety of compounds found within Indica is reported to have mental effects that are more relaxing and sedating.

Marij/huana (vs. cannabis): initially a pejorative term for cannabis derived from Mexican slang, now more commonly used to refer to dried cannabis buds, leaves and associated plant products, as well as in the conjoined term "Medical Marijuana."

Medicated: often used in lieu of the term "high" or "stoned"

NIDA: National Institute on Drug Abuse, the federal agency that currently mediates provision of cannabis to FDA-approved research studies that address drug abuse

NORML: National Organization for the Reform of Marijuana Laws. Formed in 1970 contemporaneously with the passage of the Controlled Substances Act (CSA), they are a non-profit organization missioned to legalize the responsible use of marijuana by adults, and to serve as an advocate for consumers to asure they have access to high quality marijuana that is safe, convenient, and affordable.

Phoenix Tears: a cannabis extract oil developed by Rick Simpson, using plants he originally grew in his own yard. The method for extraction is posted on his website.

Sativa: one of the main varieties of the *Cannabaceae* species originating primarily from equatorial areas of the world. The mental effects derived from this varietal are reported to be more uplifting and creativity-inducing.

Sinsemilla: "without seed", refers to the asexual cloning of plants, such that fertilization is unnecessary and a cultivar can be limited to specific female strains

Terpene: a wide variety of aromatic compounds found within cannabis and other vascular plants. These chemicals imparts the characteristic smell and flavor to cannabis, and the wide variety gives rise to an assortment of cannabis products designed to suit the user's taste inclinations. Apart from personal preferences, terpenes have demonstrated benefits for medicinal and aromatherapy purposes.

THC: abbreviation for (-)-trans-Δ9-tetrahydrocannabinol, the primary cannabinoid found in the cannabis plant and the most studied.

Tincture: an extract of oils, typically suspended in alcohol or glycerol. By using a dropper, measured amounts may be administered under the tongue or added to other products.

Vaporizing/Vaping: as an alternative to smoking, cannabis and related products may be gently heated to their boiling points producing a vapor, however, combustion does not occur. Multiple commercial products are available, similar to electronic cigarettes, with prefilled cartridges or chambers for plant material.

Introduction

What is Cannabis?

Cannabis species are ancient plants indigenous to south or central Asia and is likely one of the first plants cultivated by man. Hemp fibers, used nearly worldwide for rope, textiles and paper were likely a major reason for the spread of the plant through multiple continents, as well as the nutrient value of hemp seeds. The cannabis resin produced by the flowering plant trichomes, which includes concentrated psychoactive substances most notably in the female plant, is likely the best-known, most controversial component used in more recent times.

Cannabaceae is genus with three separate species or varieties. *Cannabis ruderalis* is a small atypical variety, mainly localized to Eastern Europe and Russia, with limited medicinal uses. *Cannabis sativa* and *Cannabis indica* are the two variants of clinical consequence. The main differences between these two species are appearance and growth characteristics. The *Cannabis sativa* and *indica* plant varietals can both contain a mixture of psychoactive and non-psychoactive substances, but most modern strains have been bred to maximize the percentage of the psychoactive substance known as THC, (-)-trans-Δ9-tetrahydrocannabinol. However, not all breeders seek to maximize the THC-induced psychoactivity. In the

United States, Great Britain and Israel, firms have developed low-THC, high-cannabidiol strains as well (Tikun Olam 2014).

The dried female flowers of the cannabis plant, commonly called simply flowers or buds, can contain up to 30% THC by weight. The term "hemp" generally refers to cannabis strains that are very low in THC, but it is also the general name for the plant fiber itself. On a federal level, hemp cannot be legally cultivated in the United States after WWII, but a number of states allow for hemp pilot studies, and eight states passed laws aimed to promote hemp agriculture. In parts of the European Union, products must contain < 0.3% dry weight or 5-10ppm THC to be considered hemp, and American states have adopted a similar standard. Although hemp does not possess the psychoactive THC, it is higher in a cannabinoid called cannabidiol (CBD). Large volumes of hemp seeds can be pressed to make hemp oil, which has nutritious omega fatty acids.

Compressed cannabis resin is referred to as "hash" or "hashish", and is generally higher in THC content than commonly available dried marijuana bud/leaf mixtures. Traditionally the hash preparation method was from the Middle East and India, using Indica varieties that produced higher amounts of resin, but modern hash products in the United States differ due to plant strain and environmental dissimilarity.

Cannabis Sativa is characterized classically by longer stalks and plants with leaves that are long and thin. Because of the long tall stalks, sativa hemp varieties are useful for fiber and are grown for this purpose in other industrialized nations. Many sativa varieties require more time to flower because they evolved in warm equatorial regions. Like indica, sativa varieties can contain a wide spectrum of THC to cannabidiol (CBD) ratios, and a variety of associated compounds as well. Common belief is that the mental effects derived from cannabis sativa use are more euphoric and uplifting.

Cannabis Indica is characterized by shorter, stalkier plants, with wider leaves and a shorter time to flowering. Native to the Middle East and Asia, this variety is the traditional source of hash and has a stronger deeper odor. The reported subjective effects of using indica varieties have been described as more sedative or fatigue-inducing.

Currently many producers categorize cannabis products based upon the strains involved:

1) Indica
2) Predominately Indica
3) Hybrid
4) Predominately Sativa
5) Sativa

It is likely that in the future a number of additional qualifiers will be applied to the characterization of cannabis products as the constituents outlined in the following chapter are further defined and isolated.

Figure 1a-c: Female flowers with magnification of crystalline resin:

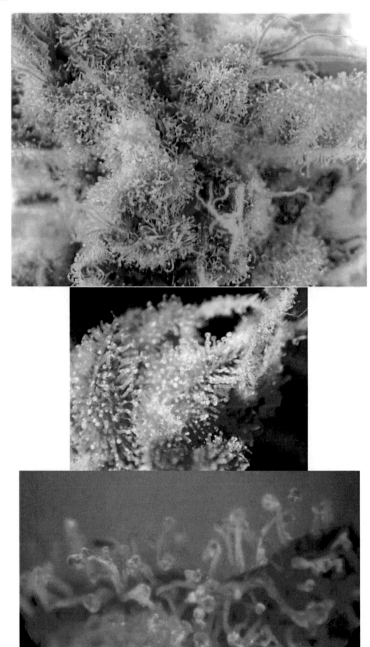

Figure 2: Cannabis indica

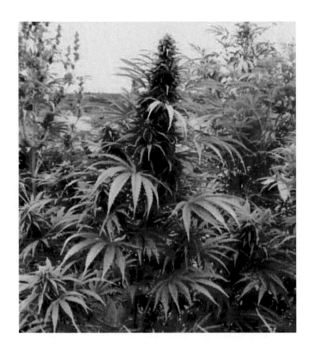

Figure 3: Cannabis sativa

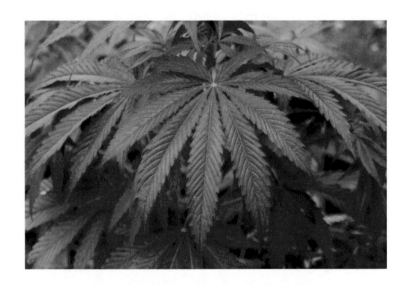

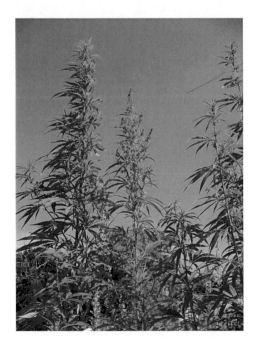

Cannabis Constituents

The cannabis plant as a whole contains hundreds of distinct compounds, which fall into chemical classes that have medically important distinctions. The most prominent and well-known terpenophenolic compounds unique to cannabis are referred to as cannabinoids or phytocannabinoids to indicate their plant origin, including tetrahydrocannabinol (THC), cannabigerol (CBG), cannabinol (CBN), cannabichromene (CBC), and cannabidiol (CBD).

To date the compounds that have been the best studied and represent the most medically important cannabinoids are THC and CBD. Each cannabis cultivar has its own unique chemical profile which can be manipulated through selective breeding and/or asexual clonal reproduction of desirable strains, called sinsemilla. Many current crops are hybridized sativa/indica strains with a wide spectrum of chemical components. Both genetic character and environment play a role in the composition of cannabinoids and the yield obtained from each harvest.

In the past, the psychoactivity of THC was the most sought-after component and genetic lineages high in CBD became increasingly rare until entities internationally began cultivating higher-CBD varieties. Contrary to the oversimplified opinion that cannabis is simply a vehicle for THC delivery, the effects of cannabinoids go far beyond THC into groundbreaking areas of molecular biology and epigenetics. Today, hundreds of strains of cannabis have been developed to genetically dispose the plant to produce particular quantities and ratios of the desired constituents. The strains may have casual names, such as diesel, AC/DC, kush and haze, but these cannabis varieties arose purposefully and systematically.

Cannabis constituent descriptions are outlined individually below, but their medical use is most often a blend, with a ratio of CBD: THC best suited to a patient's specific need.

Δ9-tetrahydrocannabinol (THC)

Identified and synthesized decades ago, Δ9-tetrahydrocannabinol, better-known as THC, is the most psychoactive of the phytocannabinoids and most likely the best-studied and commonly familiar. As the chemical responsible for the majority of the psychoactivity of the cannabis plant, it causes most of the controversy as well. In addition to its notorious mental effects, THC has multiple other medical properties through its augmentation of the endocannabinoid system discussed in a later chapter, including tempering of pain and nausea perception.

Table 1: THC structure

THC 2-D structure	THC 3-D representation

At the federally-endorsed University of Mississippi, the Potency Monitoring Project (UMPMC) analyzes samples of confiscated marijuana, "ditch weed", and hash for cannabinoid content. Samples of confiscated cannabis in the United States have revealed that the THC content had risen from 1-2% in 1980 to over 12% in 2012, with some samples surpassing 30% (Mehmedic 2010), (M. ElSohly 2014). In 2014, samples of marijuana seized in Switzerland reached a similar average of 11.5% THC (Ambach 2014). These trends give credence to the widely held belief that marijuana is "stronger" now than it was in the past, assuming that confiscated samples are representative. Given the wide range of THC in illicit samples, it could be difficult for users to predict the mental effects of use.

Figure 4: Rising Percentage of THC in Confiscated Marijuana Samples

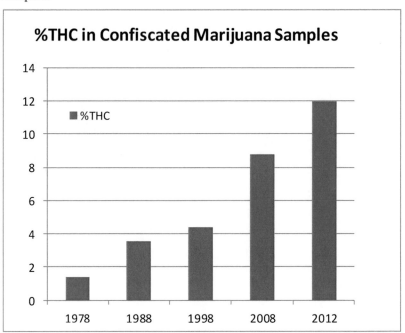

Cannabidiol (CBD)

CBD is likely the second best-studied cannabinoid as of late, after a drastic increase in research in the last decade. It lacks psychoactive effects itself and mutes the psychoactivity of THC, so a combination of THC and CBD can be used to prevent untoward mental effects of cannabis use. Because CBD has not been extensively studied as a monotherapy until very recently, it is difficult to outline the full range of benefits in humans. However, animal studies have demonstrated favorable effects for conditions such as psychiatric disorders, epilepsy, autoimmune disease, and cancer.

CBD very recently became more well-known because of its putative effects upon refractory pediatric seizure disorders such as Dravet syndrome. A growing market for predominately-CBD or CBD-only products has arisen from the promising research regarding seizure disorders as well as autoimmune disorders and cancer. A number of states have made a legal distinction between CBD and marijuana in the last couple of years, such that "marijuana" remains illegal but CBD is considered separately. These legislative efforts will expand access to this non-psychoactive medicine to patients and families even in states where cannabis is generally prohibited. CBD is available in CBD-rich oils, edibles, topicals, tinctures, and oral capsules.

Other cannabinoids

Cannabinol (CBN) is a breakdown product of THC, so is often found in cannabis products aged by time, heat and/or light. It shares some of the psychoactivity of THC, but has greater affinity for CB2 receptors, so has more effects upon the immune system. It does have some psychoactive effects, but at approximately 10% the activity of THC. Other effects are similar to its parent compound, including reduction in spasms, insomnia, and pain related to inflammation.

Interest in other minor cannabinoids has grown as well, although they typically only comprise <1% of cannabis by weight. Cannabigerol (CBG), as its name implies, is a precursor molecule for other cannabinoids, and has shown success as an anti-inflammatory (Ruhaak 2011) and antimicrobial (M. a. ElSohly 2005). In limited studies, the minor constituent cannabichromene (CBC) has shown anti-inflammatory properties as well, which appear non-receptor related, and can act synergistically with THC in mice (DeLong 2010).

Analogues of the more common cannabinoids with a propyl side chain are also found in cannabis, including CBDV (cannabidivarin) and THCV (tetrahydrocannabivarin). These compounds have similar properties to their more well-known siblings. Like CBD, cannabidivarin has antiepileptic properties and can desensitize TRPV1 channels, which makes it a potential mediator of general neuronal hyperactivity (Iannotti 2014).

THCV is of special interest because it exhibits some concentration-dependent and competitive antagonist action at CB1 and agonist action at CB2, and may act as an appetite suppressant in mice (Riedel 2009) with promising research underway for treatment of insulin-resistance. It does have psychoactivity due to activity at CB1, but has been described as milder and clearer, and does not cause hyperexcitabiltiy in animal models (J. e. McPartland 2014). Until human studies are undertaken, its full potential is unclear.

Raw forms

The naturally-occurring, sometimes called "raw" form of THC and other cannabinoids has a carboxylic acid side chain, so are often denoted as THCA, CBDA, etc. Decarboxylation into the phenolic form is required for psychotropic effects, and can occur both slowly with time, or more quickly with application of heat. The percentage of acid versus phenolic forms varies highly based on the climate in which the plant is grown. Approximately five minutes at 180-200°C is sufficient for decarboxylation, but higher heat produced during cigarette smoking achieves decarboxylation in much less time (F. Grotenhermen, Clinical Pharmakinetics of Cannabinoids 2006). The higher temperatures achieved with combustion and sometimes with manufacture will inactivate the majority of naturally-occurring volatile terpenes.

Terpenes

There is also another important class called the terpenes, aromatic compounds that impart flavor and the characteristic odor, but have less well-defined medical purposes (Clarke 2007). It has been suggested that the terpene constituents contribute to a number of effects experienced by intake of whole cannabis herb as opposed to isolated THC (J. a. McPartland 2001), which is often termed the "entourage effect." Like cannabinoids, terpenes are lipophilic, and many can cross the blood brain barrier, so it is quite feasible that they work in conjunction with other cannabinoids in the central nervous system. Many terpenes are not unique to cannabis, and can be found in other herbs such as citrus plants, rosemary, lavender, lemongrass and hops, and are known to have a variety of benefits including control of carcinogenesis, inflammation and microbial growth. In the study of aromatherapy, even small amounts of inhaled aromatics such as the terpenes can affect mood.

As an example, the terpene beta-caryophyllene is found in black pepper, basil, oregano, cinnamon, rosemary, hops, and cloves. In mice, it has been shown to be an agonist of the CB2 receptor, but its medicinal properties as a dietary cannabinoid are not fully explored (Gertsch, Beta-caryoophyllene is a dietary cannabinoid 2008).

Terpenes likely contribute to the entourage effect by providing balance to psychotropic effects. In ancient times, terpene-rich foods such as lemons, pine nuts and black pepper were used to counteract unpleasant effects of cannabis, and now with the knowledge of terpene mechanisms, these ancient practices gained merit (E. Russo 2011).

Flavonoids

Additionally, flavonoids present in other commercialized herbal preparations are also present in cannabis. A flavonoid called apigenin, better-known in chamomile, exerts anxiolytic properties by binding to central GABA receptors. The popularized flavonoid quercetin as well as a number of the known cannabinoids acts as potent antioxidant, and together they mediate a number of downstream benefits such as scavenging free radicals and inhibiting inflammation.

Apart from THC and CBD, a number of the associated phytochemicals within cannabis possess the ability to inhibit the cytochrome P450 system of the liver. In modern medicine, this must be taken into effect because of the metabolism of other exogenous prescription medications. However, the P450 system is also responsible for metabolism of carcinogen precursors to active metabolites, so inhibition of this system can lead to chemo-protection in nature. A well-studied example is the oxidation of the aflatoxin found in *Aspergillus* species into hepatotoxic metabolites.

Holistic Approach

While the cannabis plant can be broken down into several of its

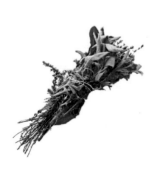

individual constituents, it would not be correct to describe the herb simply as a list of ingredients. At this time, it is likely that the "active ingredients" of a particular strain will be listed as THC and CBD percentages, but over time additional constituents may likely be quantified as well. However, it will not be possible in the near future to completely quantify the hundreds of compounds and their interactions, so the exact properties of the whole herb must be revealed over time.

In some aspects, the descriptions of cannabis varieties are reminiscent of the experience of wine consumption and the subjective experiential terms used by sommeliers. While the active ingredient, ethyl alcohol, is listed and quantified, there are other aspects to wine intake that are more difficult to quantify yet have known physiologic effects. The example below is an illustration of two wine types with the same alcohol content, but other important attributes that may not be specified on the label.

Table 2: Drawing an Anology to Wine

	Wine A	Wine B
Alcohol content	14%	14%
Grape varietal	Chardonnay	Malbec
Unlisted ingredients	Higher in sulfites	Higher in tannins
Unlisted factors	Yeast and sugar residuals	Tyramines from aging
Flavor profile	Fruity, flowery notes	Nose of cinnamon and blackberry

Considering the wine as a whole, rather than focusing on the single active ingredient, would lead one to recommend wine A for a migraineur sensitive to tannins.

Cannabis-Based Medical Therapy

While the cannabis plant has been in popular use for centuries, recent developments in the political, biochemical and medical arenas have brought the medical benefits of cannabis to the foreground of medical research. Looking back to the development of opiates, there are similarities: a plant had been cultivated for centuries for its desirable properties, the active substance was identified, extracted, modified and synthesized, then generally accepted as a medical therapy. Cannabis is earlier in this process of acceptance, and is developing in a different age of medicine where a whole herb is not as trusted as an isolated chemical created in a lab and pressed into a tablet. As our understanding of the complex interactions of chemicals within the human body changes, medical science continues to progress. Only within the last 25 years has the exact structure of THC, CBD, and their major CB1 and CB2 receptors been defined (R. Pertwee 1997). This major advance in the molecular biology of cannabinoids has launched invigorated research efforts to the therapeutic potential of this historically medicinal plant.

Cannabis-Based Medicines and US Historical Background

Cannabis has a long, conflicted history in politics, society and medicine. Physicians trained at different periods in this history are likely to have internalized various opinions and even biased education regarding how cannabis should be approached as a medication. In the early 1900's, cannabis extracts were required pharmacy stocks. The Marihuana Tax Act of 1937 changed how cannabis was regulated such that it amounted to prohibition, and therefore, made cannabis unavailable for medical treatment. The federal 1970 Controlled Substances Act then regulated marijuana as a highly addictive substance with no medical value, subject to criminal penalty. Efforts were underway throughout to end the prohibition, but research on a Schedule I substance is difficult, and conflicts arose among medical panels, organizations such as NORML, and leaders in levels of government. Societal influences such as the "War on Drugs," the AIDS epidemic and healthcare costs have also contributed to the evolving conflict, ultimately leading to the complicated and at times illogical framework currently positioned around medical cannabis today.

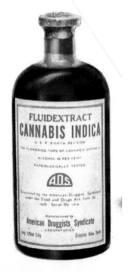

Compassionate Use Program

The "Compassionate Single Investigational New Drug Program" began in 1976 as a novel approach to the federally complex legal status of marijuana. After a glaucoma patient filed a

lawsuit contending that his marijuana use was justified, federal judge
James Washington ruled:

> ...*no adverse effects from the smoking of marijuana have*
> *been demonstrated...Medical evidence suggests that the*
> *medical prohibition is not well-founded* (The Criminal Law
> Reporter 1976)

A small core group of patients was approved to receive federally-
grown and funded marijuana cigarettes through NIDA and the
University of Mississippi, under the premise that each individual
case was receiving the material as an Investigational New Drug
(IND). Now decades old, only four surviving patients continue to
receive the metal tins packed with cigarettes. Monitoring their usage
over the years has provided some information regarding average
consumption amounts, but no formal investigational research was
undertaken on these individual patient studies with n=1. On
average, the patients consume between 6-8 grams of cannabis
bud/leaf each day, or about 6.63 pounds per year (E. e. Russo 2002).
The program received an influx of applications with the AIDS
epidemic, but was closed to new applicants in 1991.

California Proposition 215
Also called the Compassionate Use act of 1996, this was the first of
what is now a growing body of state medical cannabis laws. It was
also groundbreaking because it was enacted by voter initiative and
pressed the issue of federal vs. state rights. In California, a medical
provider can recommend cannabis for any condition in which

marijuana might be of benefit, and patients are able to both grow and smoke cannabis in a non-public setting.

Following California's lead, a number of other states enacted medical marijuana legislation, but with variations regarding regulation of home cultivation, herbal cannabis versus extracts, and the number of qualifying medical conditions. In another groundbreaking step, the people of the states of Colorado and Washington were first to "legalize" cannabis, effectively allowing for the use and regulation of cannabis in a manner similar to alcohol. Colorado first opened retail outlets January 1, 2014 (Colorado 2011) and Seattle followed in July.

Intersection of Medical and Recreational Use

The potential psychoactivity of some cannabinoids has led to both medicinal and recreational use for thousands of years, but it was not until recently that medical technology can disentangle the two areas. The psychoactivity alone however will discourage many physicians from recommending cannabis use, particularly if patients seem to be seeking the mental effects more than the medicinal benefits. The media has long portrayed users of cannabis to be mentally addled, deranged, dazed, or just lazy. Movies featuring the use of nonpsychoactive CBD in chronically ill, suffering patients are not likely to gain popularity, so the stereotype may persist. In the past, cannabis was simply considered a plant that delivered THC to get a person "stoned", and without education for both the providers and patients regarding the range of cannabinoids and their purposes, both parties may be reluctant to initiate cannabis therapy.

Misuse or abuse of healthcare industry in the United States is in the news nearly every day, and the growing medical cannabis field is unlikely to be exempt. Licensed providers who operate clinics with no function other than providing cannabis recommendations may be disposed to financial incentives. Patients with ulterior motives may find that unethical providers are apt to provide recommendations without a proper medical exam. Unfortunately, the misuse of the system reflects negatively upon the conscientious providers and patients who seek cannabis to treat existing medical conditions that have been shown objectively to benefit from cannabis.

Establishing a boundary between purely medical use and recreational use is simple for cannabinoids such as cannabidiol, but more difficult for products containing psychoactive cannabinoids. On the contrary, in states such as Colorado and Washington, recreational cannabis is available without seeking medical attention so the boundary is drawn outside of the doctor-patient relationship. Patients who are comfortable asking about medical cannabis may have previous experience with recreational marijuana use, and providers may feel as though medical cannabis is simply an excusable route of obtaining recreational cannabis. Some providers may have had negative experiences with patients "seeking" pain medications, and translate the experience to cannabis patients as well. In one study of Canadian HIV-positive patients, 80% of patients using medicinal cannabis also continued using cannabis recreationally (Furler 2004). A much larger survey of over 4000 medical cannabis users in California revealed that nearly 90% used daily or near-daily inhaled medical cannabis (O'Connell 2007), which would may preclude the need for additional recreational cannabis.

Ultimately, a black-and-white line may not be possible. The art of medical practice requires evaluation of gray areas on a regular basis, and providers of cannabis therapy must follow ethical principles in this area as well.

What Providers and Patients Need to Know about Cannabis Legislation

At this time, 20 states and the District of Columbia have legislation supporting medical cannabis use, two states for non-medical use, and 11 states have legislation passed or in process considering CBD separately from other marijuana prohibition. Because of the variability in state laws, licensed providers are wise to investigate the laws of the state(s) in which they practice. Many laws specify cannabis quantities in grams or ounces, which refers to the dried plant material rather than other forms such as extracts and edibles, which further complicates interpretation of state regulations.

The intricacies of cannabis legislation can be difficult enough for trade experts to understand, so it is likely that patients will have difficulties understanding how to use medical cannabis in a legally appropriate fashion. Some rough guidelines can answer some of the most common patient questions without delving into formal legal advice:

- What medical problems is medical cannabis used for?
- Can I travel out-of-state with my medicine?
- Can I order products like hemp oil online? What cannabis products can be shipped?
- Can I grow my own plants at home?
- What forms of cannabis are medical? Can this be smoked, or vaporized?
- Can I drive after I take my medicine?
- Who can give the medicine to patients like children or disabled adults?
- Is there a difference between retail/recreational cannabis and medical cannabis?
- Do I have to carry a cannabis license?
- Will my work drug screen make me lose my job?

Patients accustomed to receiving a prescription and proceeding to a retail pharmacy will also encounter some questions. Rather than a prescription where the provider proscribes the exact dose and timing, cannabis dosing is not often so black-and-white. Different patients respond differently to its effects, and individual titrations are often required to achieve the optimal dose and timing. At dispensaries, the personnel assisting patients with this process may range from budtenders with no formal education to clinicians to pharmacists, and this contrast from the typical retail pharmacy may raise patient questions as well regarding who is directing their care.

Federally, any form of plant-based cannabis remains schedule I, which has led to numerous court battles regarding state vs. federal conflicts. It remains unclear how federally-based institutions such as CMS and the DEA will respond to DEA-licensed providers who also choose to write cannabis recommendation letters. In California and the rest of the Ninth Circuit, the 2007 appeals case of *Conant v. McCaffrey* does protect providers under the First Amendment to make medical cannabis recommendations, but other districts have no such case precedents and the case does not protect the dispensaries themselves. As yet, there have not been widespread DEA license revocations in medical cannabis states, but some reports have recently arisen regarding providers receiving warnings from the DEA in Massachusetts (Lazar 2014).

Medical Society Positions on Medical Cannabis

Providers likely formed different opinions about cannabis during the era of strict prohibition than they would form today. After various states have passed diverse cannabis regulations, physician opinion may vary regionally as well. Physicians in a specialty such as oncology may have differing opinions than a sports medicine specialist, based on their daily experiences. An unfortunate byproduct of the political attitudes toward cannabis is that the natural endocannabinoid system and its manipulation is not freely taught in medical school curriculums, so the knowledge base of providers varies as well. This patchwork of influences leads to heterogeneity in provider attitudes, and the messages they communicate to patients.

In the face of contradictory opinions regarding a controversial subject such as cannabis, respected organizations such as the

American Medical Association (AMA) and American College of Physicians (ACP) may offer useful information and guidance.

Reports from the AMA in 2009, and updated in 2013, addressed both the medical use and the social effects of cannabis in policies H-95.992, H-95.995 and H-95.98. To summarize, the AMA supported approaches to conduct more rigorous scientific evaluations regarding the medicinal values of cannabis. In that context, they recognized that the schedule I classification of cannabis hinders research efforts, and in 2009 they endorsed reclassification for this purpose. The vote reached in 2009 does represent a reversal of a long-held position that marijuana should remain classified as schedule I, which was previously reaffirmed in 2001. From the executive summary of the Council on Science and Public Health (CSAPH) report in 2009:

> *The future of cannabis-based medicine lies in the rapidly evolving field of botanical drug substance development, as well as the design of molecules that target various aspects of the endocannabinoid system. To the extent that rescheduling marijuana out of schedule one will benefit this effort, such a move can be supported.* (American Medical Association 2009)

They also recommended the formulation of a more comprehensive national drug policy, particularly to address issues of adolescent drug use. In 2013, they did retain language that "cannabis is a dangerous drug and as such is a public health concern", as well as opposition to widespread, undifferentiated legalization.

Similarly, the American College of physicians supports increased funding and research into the area of medicinal cannabis. Their position paper in 2008 included appetite stimulation, nausea relief, neurological and movement disorders, glaucoma, and pain relief as potential medical uses. They also urged:

> ...an evidence-based review of marijuana's status as a Schedule I controlled substance to determine whether it should be reclassified to a different schedule. This review should consider the scientific findings regarding marijuana's safety and efficacy in some clinical conditions as well as evidence on the health risks associated with marijuana consumption, particularly in its crude smoked form. (American College of Physicians 2008)

What do other physicians think about medical marijuana? A recent survey by WebMD asked over 1500 physicians, with the majority of physicians indicating that it help with certain conditions (69%) and that it should be a medical option for patients (67%). Oncologists, who are likely more familiar with cannabis-based medicines, had even higher responses at 82% (Rappold 2014).

New Approaches to Medical Cannabis Utility

Generally, the concept of cannabis as a medicine has been well-accepted in the ancient as well as more recent medical society. The historical perspective of cannabis is addressed expertly in other books (see author Ethan Russo), so will not be covered here in detail; instead, presentation of how the medical cannabis field has changed in recent decades.

Contemporaneously, the delivery of healthcare in America has experienced significant changes as well. Partially due to cost factors as well as other societal issues, many Americans are turning to complementary and alternative medicine. In 1990, one third of Americans used some form of alternative medicine, which nearly doubled over the following decade (Su 2011). This resurgence in alternative, holistic, homeopathic and/or naturalistic medicine is concomitant with the acceptance of using herbal preparations such as cannabis as medicines.

Cannabis-based medications are not often used first-line, as monotherapy, or to replace traditional medical treatment; rather, as adjuncts to conditions that are difficult to treat with conventional medicines, or in patients who have had difficulties with conventional treatments. A collection of neurologic disorders falls in this category, as well as terminal illnesses such as cancer and AIDS. The limited medical modalities that attempt to treat the recalcitrant underlying medical pathophysiology often carry a heavy side effect burden for patients and their caregivers, so seeking alternative treatments is a natural inclination.

Symptom-based medications such as opiates have been in use for decades, but their side effect profile is also taxing: including lethargy, nausea, constipation, addiction, and overdose. So pervasive have the negative effects of opiates been upon American society, that counties in California have filed a lawsuit against several opiate manufacturers for misleading medical providers about opiate safety (http://bit.ly/11Hxf8q). Further, a study released online by JAMA in August 2014 indicated that states with medical marijuana laws had a nearly 25% reduction in annual opioid overdose death rate as compared to states without such laws, and that the reduction in fatalities grew year-by-year following legislation passage (Bachhuber 2014). Also in 2014, the well-known opiate hydrocodone will be re-classified from schedule III to schedule II, reflecting the increased scrutiny on American opiate use.

While the mood-altering properties of cannabis are common knowledge, what has not been well-known until recently is that cannabinoids have disease-modification benefits related to neurologic and inflammatory pathophysiology. As a result, cannabinoids have a unique medicinal profile insofar as they can simultaneously alter disease pathology, offer immediate symptom reduction, and pose little risk for serious deleterious side effects.

The Endocannabinoid System

In medicine, understanding first the normal physiologic process is essential to understanding how it can be manipulated. A variety of endocannabinoid molecules, chemically similar to compounds in cannabis, exist naturally within the nervous system of humans and other mammals. The term "endocannabinoid" arose retroactively after the elucidation of their similarity to phytocannabinoids, but these chemicals are endogenous to mammalian biology and despite the name, should not be confused with exogenous cannabinoids derived from cannabis. Initially perplexing, the designation does logically correlate with the pharmacologic history of opium, where an cultivated plant (poppy) produces chemicals that mimic the action of endogenous molecules (endorphins, e.g. endo-morphine), that bind to existing receptors (μ receptor). Among the five endocannabinoids identified in the 1990's, two have emerged as the most functionally important: anandamide or *N*-arachidonoylethanolamine (AEA) and 2-arachidonoylglycerol (2-AG), each pictured below:

Anandamide

2-Arachidonylglycerol (2-AG)

Other human endocannabinoids include 2-arachidonylglyceryl ether (noladin ether), O-arachidonoyl-ethanolamine (virodhamine), and N-arachidonoyl-dopamine (NADA). Based upon the common root - arachido-, the similar chemical nature of these chemicals is apparent. Arachidonic acid, at times abbreviated ARA or AA, is a fatty acid similar to dietary omega-6 fatty acids.

Because they are produced on-demand, endocannabinoids differ from classical neurotransmitters which are stored in vesicles, so they are often termed neuromodulators instead. Endocannabinoids are produced through depolarization-initiated, intracellular-calcium mediated phospholipase cleavage of precursors in the lipid cell membrane. In some disease states, and in response to physiologic stress such as neuronal damage, levels of endocannabinoids are increased by cleaving the membrane precursors as needed. Studies suggest that an increase in endocannabinoid levels facilitates recovery from oxidative stress, free radical damage, and the subsequent inflammation produced by apoptosis.

In nerve tissues, endocannabinoids function as retrograde neuromodulators in a complex feedback system.

Figure 5: High-level Depiction of Forward Neurotransmission
"Chemical synapse schema cropped" by user:Looie496 created file, US NIH, National Institute on Aging created original - http://www.nia.nih.gov/Alzheimers/Publications/UnravelingtheMystery/. Licensed under Public domain via Wikimedia Commons

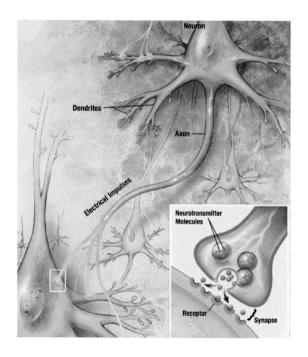

Figure 6: Simplified endocannabinoid Neuromodulatory Cycle

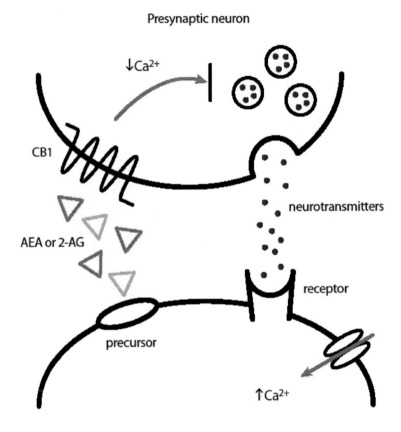

In vivo, AEA is quickly inactivated enzymatically by the fatty acid amide hydrolase (FAAH). AEA can be potentiated by inhibition of the FAAH catalytic enzyme (Hwang J 2010) or by methylation modification of the anandamide molecule to impede FAAH action.

2-AG is broken down by monoglyceride lipase primarily, as well as other enzymes.

Sites of Exogenous Cannabinoid Action

THC and many of its derivatives are agonists at the CB1 and CB2 receptors in tissues where those receptors are expressed. Intake of THC systemically, in the amounts used in therapeutic and recreational doses, causes activation of these receptors that is more widespread and nonspecific than the subtle modulatory effects of natural endocannabinoids.

The mechanism of action of CBD remained unclear for years because it only showed weak affinity to the known CB receptors and actually has some inhibitory effects for CB1 and CB2 agonists at the receptor. Recent research suggests that one of CBD's main mechanisms of action is inhibiting FAAH-mediated hydrolysis of AEA. By delaying AEA breakdown, mean levels of AEA are increased. CBD is also an inhibitor of p450-mediated oxidation of THC so can prolong the action of THC in vivo.

Figure 7: Sites of Cannabinoid Action

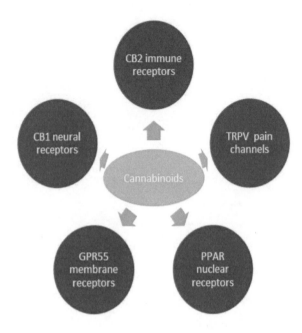

Connection to Dietary Fatty Acids and Supplements

A variety of fatty acids are required for normal cell membrane functioning, and "essential" fatty acids are those of the body cannot synthesize, but are necessary for health. In humans, the two essential fatty acids are alpha linoleic acid (ALA) and linoleic acid, both of which belong to the omega fatty acid family. Intake of omega (ω) fatty acids leads to modification in the mammal to eicosanoids (then prostaglandins, leukotrienes) and arachidonic acid—a component of the endocannabinoids AEA and 2-AG.

Docosahexaenoic acid (DHA) and eicosapentaenoic acid (EPA) are polyunsaturated ω3 fatty acids made from ALA and found in fish oil, canola oil, flaxseed, walnuts and wild rice. Normally found in high concentrations in neuronal membranes, low levels of these fatty acids have been linked to depression as well as cardiovascular disease. When these molecules are esterified with ethanolamide, they display endocannabinoid similarities such as activating CBRs and breakdown by FAAH catalysis (Brown 2010).

Considering the high amounts in neural tissue and the demands of a developing brain, polyunsaturated fatty acid supplementation was theorized to support mental development in infants, and led to DHA and arachidonic acid-enriched baby formulas (Birch 2007).

Other dietary compounds can affect endocannabinoids as well. Naturally-occurring unsaturated fatty acids in chocolate, Noleoylethanolamine and N-linoleoylethanolamine do not directly bind to the CB1 receptor, however they do inhibit the FAAH-mediated breakdown of AEA in rat brain, indirectly increasing AEA levels (di Tomaso 1996).

Hemp oil contains essential fatty acids as well as the desired 3:1 ratio of ω6:3 fatty acids. Studies regarding the health benefits of fish and other oils revealed that the ω6 and ω3 fatty acids are best consumed in a 2-3:1 ratio, which is uncommon in the Western diet, so supplements have been developed that enhance this ratio.

Together, the fatty acid nature of the endocannabinoids and the research regarding fatty acid intake suggest that indeed measured dietary intake of essential fatty acids is beneficial for the delicate interplay amongst cell membrane function in the ubiquitous endocannabinoid system.

Exogenous Phytocannabinoids

Pictured below are the two primary cannabinoids found in cannabis: THC and CBD. These molecules exert their effects by enhancing the endocannabinoid system. THC binds to both the CB1 and CB2 receptors, and CBD hinders the hydrolysis of AEA, so together they can augment natural endocannabinoid functioning in a synergistic fashion. Other phytocannabinoids are discussed in the Cannabis Constituents section.

THC	CBD

A non-cannabis plant compound has also been discovered to have cannabinomimetic activity at CB2—N-akyl amides from *Echinacea*/purple coneflower (Gertsch 2006). Ongoing discoveries of such as this may lead to further research into related plant compounds that affect the endocannabinoid system.

Synthetic Cannabinoids

After the discovery of both the natural endocannabinoid structure as well as their receptors, scientists began investigations as to how the system could be modified to achieve specific effects. Laboratory modifications of cannabinoids can alter their affinity for CB receptors, interfere with the actions of other cannabinoids, and alter hydrolytic kinetics. These synthetic or modified cannabinoids are not generally purposed for medicinal use at this time, but they are quite useful in laboratory investigations and research regarding endocannabinoid signaling pathways.

Back in 1977, laboratories began experimenting with synthetic enantiomers of THC and cannabidiol in the + configuration, that were dubbed "abnormal" or abn-THC, abn-CBD (Adams 1977).

They noted that abn-CBD had vasodilatory effects, without causing behavior changes in the laboratory dogs. Many years later, this observation is now believed to be related to a proposed new cannabinoid receptor, GPR18, which mediates the vasodilatory effects of AEA and abn-CBD (Penumarti and Abdel-Rahman 2014).

Another synthetic cannabinoid molecule was developed as an inhibitor rather than an agonist. Given that cannabinoids typically induce appetite, it might follow that blockade of the cannabinoid system may be useful for weight loss. SR141716A is an antagonist at CB1 receptors, and did indeed show appetite suppression in mice. As an investigational medication, it was called rimonabant/Acomplia and underwent trials in Europe which did show weight loss.

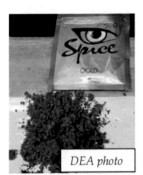

DEA photo

Unfortunately untoward mental effects in humans resulted, which underscores the importance of the endocannabinoid system in normal human physiology.

Synthetic cannabinoids have also been manufactured for recreational use, and in recent years substances called K2 and "spice" have emerged in the US market. Many of these "designer" drugs are CB1 agonists, but are structurally dissimilar to natural THC. The increased incidence of adverse effects related to these illicit substances is partially related to very potent activation of the CB1 receptor, but also multiple effects in the other neurotransmitter systems such as serotonin (Seely 2013).

Medicinal Cannabinoids: Mechanism of Action

The elucidation of exogenous and endocannabinoid molecular structure, along with their receptor targets, has led to a great deal of research on the mechanisms through which the cannabinoids work in the human body. At least two cannabinoid receptors have been well-defined: CB1 and CB2. They are the most abundant G-protein coupled receptor in the CNS, yet were relatively unknown until the 1990's when research volume regarding cannabinoids skyrocketed. The CB1 and CB2 receptors are both G-protein-linked and stereoselective, but display disparate properties in other aspects.

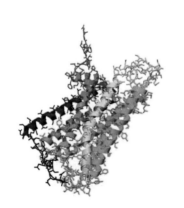

CB1 receptors are found primarily on neurons within the central and peripheral nervous system, but also in smaller concentrations other cells such as lymphocytes, retinal and endocrine cells. CB1 receptors activation leads to the downstream psychoactive effects of cannabis.

Figure 8: Structure of the CB1 receptor

Source: P21554 CNR1_HUMAN Cannabinoid receptor 1 OS=Homo sapiens GN=CNR1 PE=1
SV=1Morten Kallberg, Haipeng Wang, Sheng Wang, Jian Peng, Zhiyong Wang, Hui Lu & Jinbo Xu.
Template-based protein structure modeling using the RaptorX web server. Nature Protocols, 7(8):
1511-1522, 2012. Public domain.

CB2 receptors are distributed differently within human tissues, concentrated in the immune system and the glia that support the CNS. Knowing the distribution of this receptor, it is logical that activation does not induce psychoactive effects; rather, immunomodulation. The THC molecule, AEA, 2-AG and synthetic analogs can activate either cannabinoid receptor at low concentrations.

CBD has not been shown to activate either the CB1 or CB2 receptor with significant affinity. Recent work has shown that the lipophilic endocannabinoids bind to fatty acid binding proteins within the cell cytoplasm and are then catalyzed by fatty acid amide hydrolase (FAAH). CBD appears to indirectly increase AEA levels by inhibiting FAAH (Bisogno 2001).

In vivo, the complex interactions amongst endocannabinoids and exogenous cannabinoids cannot be oversimplified to a linear process. As neuromodulators, cannabinoids typically exhibit an inhibitory feedback effect upon the neurotransmitter released at the presynaptic terminal. Some neurotransmitters are suppressive and others are excitatory, so the net effect may in fact be upregulation. The neural pathways of the mammalian brain are not simply excitatory or inhibitory either, and these tissues may express different ratios of receptors, so the overall effect of cannabinoids upon the CNS is incredibly complex. The widespread distribution of CB and non-CB receptors makes manipulation of a single area much more difficult. Clearly the pharmaceutical potential is also vast, so in the future highly specific pharmaceutical modulators of the endocannabinoid system are sure to develop.

Figure 9: Immunohistochemical Staining for the CB1 Receptor in a Sagittal Section of Mouse Brain

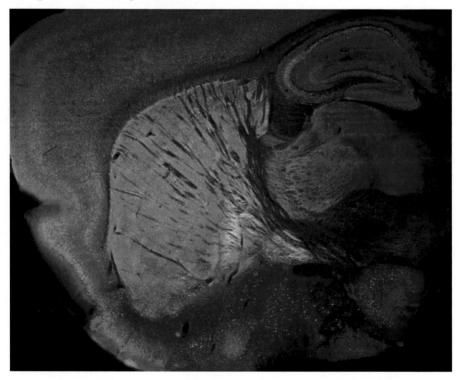

Source: National Institutes of Health (NIH) Creator: Margaret I. Davis Date Added: 5/24/2012. Image was taken with a Zeiss Lumar stereomicroscope. Public domain.

Figure 10: Sites of CB1 Receptors

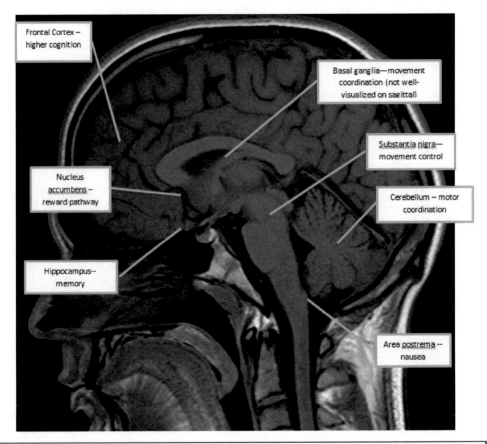

Figure 11: Mechanism of endocannabinoids at nerve terminals

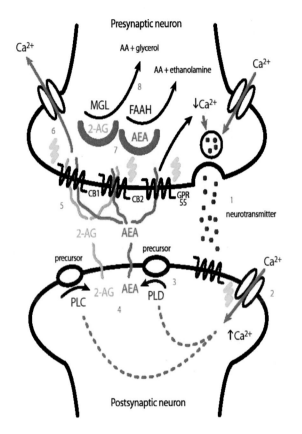

1. The cycle begins with the release of a neurotransmitter from the activated presynaptic neuron

2. Crossing the synapse, the neurotransmitter binds to receptors on the postsynaptic membrane and causes depolarization and opening of calcium channels

3. The influx of calcium then triggers a cascade of events which leads to phospholipase-induced cleavage of endocannabinoid precursors in the cell membrane

4. AEA and 2-AG are released into the cleft and diffuse to the presynaptic terminal.

5. There, they bind to the G-protein coupled cannabinoid receptors CB1 and CB2, as well as non-CB receptors GPR55 and TRPV1 for AEA

6. Decreased intracellular calcium levels result, resulting in negative feedback to step 1

7. Internalized AEA and 2-AG bind to intracellular fatty acid binding proteins

8. AEA is broken down into ethanolamine and arachidonic acid by FAAH, and 2-AG is broken down into glycerol and arachidonic acid by MGL

Elucidation of non-CB Receptors

GPR55

The CB1 and CB2 receptors were characterized in the 1960's by Dr. Mechoulam's renowned research laboratory. Another receptor, GPR55, was more recently cloned in 1999. Despite its widespread presence throughout the CNS, it remained an orphan receptor until more recently when it was noted that it shared sequence similarity to the binding region of cannabinoid receptors (D. Baker 2006). AEA as well as THC binds to the GPR55 receptor, and 2-AG can be interconverted to GPR55's primary ligand L-α-lysophosphatidylinositol (LPI) (Zhao 2013). Similar to its actions at CB receptors, CBD is more likely a GPR55 antagonist (H. a. Sharir 2010). Together, the evidence supports that GPR55 does play a role in the interdependencies of the cannabinoid system, with more research underway.

TRPV1
Also known as the Vanilloid Receptor 1 (VR1), the transient receptor potential vanilloid (TRPV1) receptor channel is activated in response to tissue irritants such as heat, decreased pH and exogenous capsaicin "heat". Mediating sensory nociception, activation of TRPV1 causes calcium ion influx and a subsequent burning sensation. However, chronic activation of the receptor leads to a paradoxical desensitization. THC and AEA also activate TRPV1, and this activation leads to phosphorylation and ion influx. CBD and CBDV, on the other hand, desensitize the receptor in vitro much like capsaicin does (Bisogno 2001) and may prove therapeutic in arthritis, neuropathic pain, and diseases of neuronal hyperexcitability (Iannotti 2014).

PPARs
Within the cell, cannabinoids also interact with peroxisome proliferator activated receptors (PPARs). These nuclear receptors

cause downstream binding to DNA promoter sequences to enhance gene transcription. The PPAR receptor family regulates lipid metabolism, and fatty acids activate the receptors in what could be a feedback mechanism. By inhibiting fatty acid hydrolase, CBD increases intracellular levels of fatty acids that bind to PPARγ such as AEA, linoleic acid, arachidonic acid, and EPA (J. a. Berger 2002). Recalling the names of the endocannabinoids and their relation to fatty acids, it follows that endocannabinoids have direct influence at PPARs as well. It is possible that other cannabinoids directly bind to PPAR, but it is not yet clear if PPAR activation is direct or indirect (Sun 2007). The FDA approved fibrates and thiazolidinediones (such as pioglitazone) for insulin sensitization, and later it was discovered that their mechanism of action was PPARα and PPARγ activation, respectively. Given the extent of diabetes and related metabolic disorders, this area has enormous pharmaceutical potential.

5-HT$_{1a}$

Taking into account that cannabis has been used for centuries to control pain and nausea, it may come as no surprise that cannabinoids can have effects upon the serotonin system and its 5-HT receptors. Dr. Ethan Russo has long recommended that cannabis should be applied to migraine therapy (E. Russo 1998), and in 2005 demonstrated that CBD has agonist effects at 5-HT$_{1a}$ receptors (E. e. Russo 2005). In addition to headache, serotonergic effects are being considered with regards to neuromodulation in the serotonergic basal ganglia (Espejo-Porras, et al. 2013), central nausea (Rock 2012), and stroke neuroprotection (Mishima 2005).

Mental Effects of Cannabinoids

Generally, a number of medical terms have been used to describe the effects of cannabis use: relaxation, intoxication, memory impairment, time distortion, increased appetite, dysphoria, euphoria, reduced concentration, reduced reaction time, dry mouth, tachycardia, conjunctival injection, hyperactivity, heightened attentiveness, depersonalization, dizziness, confusion, flushing, somnolence, vision changes, and disorientation.

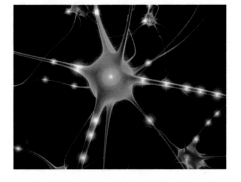

In addition to familiar medical terminology, patients may report a wider variety of colloquial terms regarding the mental alterations of cannabis: chill, dreamy, floating, heaviness, peaceful, whole-body, relaxation, euphoria, "body" effect, head rush, social effect, uplifting, chatty, creative, focus, laid-back, foggy, "couch lock", attentive, buzz, hilarity, or time-expansion.

The range of symptoms experienced by cannabis user will vary based upon the components of cannabis contained within the product used, the route of administration, the metabolism of the individual user, as well as their environment and mental mindset. It may be difficult then to predict accurately how any one individual patient may react to medicinal cannabis, so generally beginning with a small initial dose and titrating upward very slowly is advisable. To be safe, naiive users may find that a safe, comfortable environment with known, trusted adults is the best setting to trial first doses of medical cannabis. Beginning with a low dose of psychoactive constituents is also advisable, to avoid inadvertent over-intensity of symptoms. A number of studies have shown that a balance of CBD can ameliorate some of the negative effects of unopposed THC (Niesink 2013), including memory loss at the hippocampus (Englund 2013).

A phenomenon known as Acute Cannabis psychosis has been described, where patients who had consumed large amounts of cannabis in a short time-frame became suddenly confused, delusional, labile, amnestic, and paranoid, then recovered with residual deficit after cannabis abstinence. This does not likely represent a primary psychiatric disorder, rather, an expected effect of large cannabis doses.

Observationally, it is often found that users can become tolerant to the unpleasant side effects relatively quickly, while preserving therapeutic effect. Because most cannabis studies are 12 weeks or less, it is difficult to quantity long-term tolerance. It is reasonable to surmise that CB receptors, if continually activated, would undergo down-regulation over time, but further study is needed to evaluate the process.

Users may tend to have a preference for one strain of cannabis over another. There is no objective evidence to demonstrate that these effects are supported by molecular biology except by accounting for THC and CBD, but after understanding the multiple active components of cannabis it is possible the lesser cannabinoids and terpenes could account for these effects.

Table 3: Subjective Differences between sativa and indica strains of cannabis

	Sativa	Indica
Subjective Effects	Euphoria	Analgesia
	Energy	Sleep
Conditions Where One Strain Preferred	Weight loss	Nonmigraine Headaches
	Recreational Use	Neuropathy
		Seizures

Source: (Pearce 2014)

Treatment

In cases of over-ingestion of cannabis, where the product consumed is known, there is likely little medical danger in overdose as outlined in the Safety Profile section below. Often a quiet, calming environment is reassuring to anxious or paranoid patients. If symptoms are severe, with psychotic or other dangerous tendencies, administration of benzodiazepines in a medical setting may be effective in reducing agitation until effects of THC wear off. Orally-ingested THC does undergo significant first-pass metabolism in the liver to a psychoactive metabolite 11-OH-THC, so prompt gut decontamination may be of some benefit in reducing the duration of symptoms.

In cases where decreased mental acuity and/or paranoia make it difficult to ascertain what substances the user may have consumed, medical attention is the most prudent approach.

Safety Profile

Within cannabis literature, it is nearly ubiquitously reported that marijuana alone has never caused a human fatality. Wayne Hall at the National Drug and Alcohol Research center in Australia has reported in a number of publications that there have been no confirmed cases of cannabis overdose, and the estimated lethal dose for humans extrapolated from animal studies is so high that it cannot be achieved by users (W. Hall 1995).

The FDA-approved medication dronabinol, consisting of Δ9-THC, indicates on the label that the estimated lethal human dose of intravenous dronabinol is 30 mg/kg (FDA rev 2004). Quantifying the LD50 of cannabis in humans has not been demonstrated, and the coexistence of other substances such as cocaine or heroin further confounds the causality in postmortem cases. A possible explanation is a paucity of receptors in the brain stem of humans, saving the overdosed patient from the respiratory depression seen in other overdoses such as opiates (F. Grotenhermen, Cannabinoids and the Endocannabinoid System 2006). Before extrapolating this observation into a blanket statement regarding the safety of cannabis, further investigation is warranted.

The LD50 value, which is the gross single dose of a substance that causes lethality in 50% of test animals, is an informative piece of data however it does not put this dose into the context of a therapeutic dose. With many prescription drugs, a therapeutic index is more useful to determine the overall safety of a particular substance. The therapeutic index is calculated by dividing the median toxic dose by the median effective dose, so the smaller the number, the more hazardous the medication.

A narrow therapeutic index is defined by the FDA as a less than 2-fold difference between median lethal and median effective dose, or between minimum toxic and minimum effective concentrations in the blood. Commonly used medications within this category include digoxin, lithium and phenytoin. Using digoxin as an example, therapeutic blood levels are approximately 0.8-2.0 ng/mL, and the toxic level is approximately 2.4 ng/mL, producing a therapeutic index of about 1.7.

For illicit or non-FDA approved substances, it is difficult to calculate a therapeutic index. In these cases, a safety ratio is often used, where Safety ratio = ratio of toxic dose to desired effective dose. Again, the smaller the number, the more risky the substance. The estimated fatal human dose of THC is between 15-70 grams. Starting with a common single dose of 20mg, this would translate into 750-3500

doses. These values are intrinsically difficult to calculate, but the
figure below depicts some estimated numbers (Gable 2004):

Figure 12: Safety ratios of commonly abused psychoactive drugs

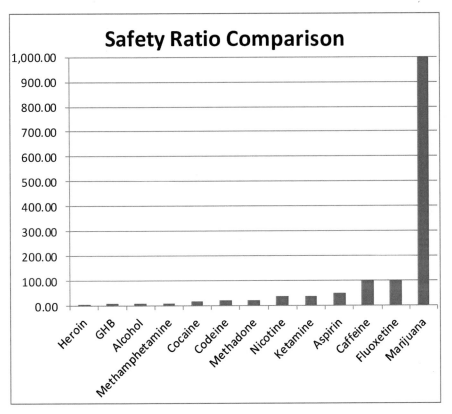

The historical safety of cannabis products preceded the development
of synthetic and other highly concentrated forms of THC. Therefore,
it is wise to carefully study which substance exactly as being
consumed, as well as the route of administration and other
underlying medical conditions when considering the overall safety of
cannabis. The recent manufacture of illicit "synthetic" products may

lead one to believe that synthetic cannabis is unsafe; however, the chemical structure of "synthetic" marijuana such as K2 is dissimilar to the natural form so the potency and metabolism is different. Fortunately with use of medicinal and other regulated products as well as careful cannabis cultivation, both patients and their medical providers are better informed regarding the active chemicals contained within cannabis products they consume.

Regardless of the known safety profile, cannabis and its related medicinal derivatives must be stored in a safe manner and labeled accurately as to avoid accidental ingestion, particularly for children.

Metabolism of Cannabinoids

After initial absorption and distribution into the bloodstream, plasma levels drop as cannabinoids distribute into highly vascularized and lipophilic tissues. Over time, cannabinoids redistribute back into the bloodstream, often causing perplexing fluctuations in blood levels. Because they are lipophilic, cannabinoids require extensive chemical modification to be eliminated.

The major modifications take place through oxidation in the hepatic cytochrome p450 system, with subsequent hydroxylation and glucoronidation. Orally consumed cannabinoids undergo significant first-pass hepatic metabolism through this mechanism. Some major metabolites produced are 11-OH-THC, THC-COOH and their glucoronidated and fatty-acid conjugated forms. Both THC and CBD are primarily metabolized through the CYP2C9 and CYP3A4 p450 subsets, which affects metabolism of other cannabinoids as well as other exogenous medications, as listed in the Cautions: Interactions section (Jiang 2011) (Watanabe 2007). Due to this first-pass liver effect, oral ingestion of THC leads to increased levels of 11-OH-THC compared to inhalation. 11-OH-THC has prolonged psychoactive effects at the CB1 receptor, so oral ingestion leads to more sustained mental status alteration.

THC	11-OH-THC

The lipophilic forms that have distributed into the body tissues are slow to re-diffuse from the body fat back into the plasma, which can result in metabolites appearing in the urine for days after exposure. Researchers have proposed that the ratio of the THC-COOH metabolite to THC can be used to estimate the elapsed time from THC exposure (Huestis 1992) and attempts to validate this research are still underway to provide guidance regarding legal matters such as driving under the influence (MA Huestis 2006). Unfortunately, there is no linear or predictable relationship amongst the time of exposure, plasma levels, degree of intoxication, or excretion. The mean terminal half-life of THC is estimated to be 30 hours but can vary widely.

Metabolized THC is excreted into the water-based bodily fluids of urine, saliva and sweat in smaller amounts compared to fecal elimination. Lipophilic free THC is completely reabsorbed by the renal tubules, so only conjugated metabolites appear in the urine.

Drug testing

The chemical detected most commonly in urinary drug tests is THC-COOH. Because of the complex metabolism of THC and variability amongst users, it is often difficult to predict how long a urine drug test will remain positive. A variety of researchers have found that 3 to 5 days is most common, however reports of persistence for weeks to months are not uncommon (F. Grotenhermen, Clinical Pharmakinetics of Cannabinoids 2006). This is likely due to the distribution of cannabis metabolite into bodily compartments at various time points. While the medicolegal aspects of cannabis drug testing is outside the scope of this book, providers recommending cannabis-based medicines likely have questions regarding detection of cannabinoids for medical and other practical reasons.

Because of its biochemical structure, CBD and its related compounds are not detected by traditional urine drug testing (Tsai 2007). Dronabinol, structurally identical to naturally- occurring

THC, undergoes the same metabolic process and is indistinguishable from illicit THC in a urine drug test. However, the presence of other cannabinoids naturally occurring in herbal cannabis, such as THCV, is a sign that a drug test was not positive due to dronabinol alone.

The Substance Abuse and Mental Health Services Administration (SAMSHA) oversees with eating federally regulated drug testing programs. They define both what constitutes a screening versus confirmatory test, as well as the cutoff level that defines a positive result. Effective 2010, the immunoassay initial testing cut off was set at 50 ng/mL, a reduction from the previous 100 ng/mL (Substance Abuse and Mental Health Services Administration 2010). The cutoff for confirmatory testing drops to 15 ng/mL, so this level is often used as a reference point in research studies.

SAMHSA also has guidelines in place for testing and reporting of sample adulteration. Widely available on the Internet, kits containing adulterants are marketed to persons wishing to mask positive urine drug screening tests. Among these methods, oxidizing agents can be used to significantly reduce the amount of THC-COOH detectable in the urine (Paul 2004).

Legally rigorous detection methods for THC metabolites in other bodily fluids are still under investigation. Point-of-care sweat and saliva detection offers an obvious advantage to urine collection, but technology has yet to meet the stringent error rates required from a medicolegal perspective.

Common Cannabis-Based Medications

The Entourage Effect

It is a common observation in clinical use that whole plant/extract oil use is often more subjectively efficacious than single isolated plant or synthetic cannabinoids such as dronabinol. This is dubbed the "entourage" effect, and over time what began as frequent subjective reports has been bourne out in the objective analysis of cannabis constituents. The interplay of the well-known cannabinoids THC, CBD, CBV, CBC and terpenes in humans has not been decisively established, but the mechanisms of action demonstrated in the laboratory makes it clear that multiple interactions are at play. While some constituents may have a synergistic effect, it is also likely that the balance of chemicals can mitigate side effects. For instance, cannabidiol is an antagonist of CB1 and CB2 agonists and inhibits the metabolism of THC to its long-acting psychoactive metabolite 11-OH-THC, so can ameliorate possible unpleasant mind-altering effects of THC. While THC, CBD and a small number of other cannabinoids have been the most extensively studied as single agents, the effects of the other 400 phytochemicals have been encompassed, and contribute to the difference in subjective effects between whole-plant and isolated extracts.

The Extract Movement

The detriments of inhaling a combustion product have long been cited as an objective medical reason to avoid cannabis use. To avoid smoking, cannabinoids have been extracted from the plant matter through a variety of methods including hydrocarbons, oils, carbon dioxide, and alcohol to produce tinctures and oils.

One of the more famous oils was pioneered by Rick Simpson from Canada, who developed "Phoenix Tears" after struggling with conventional medications for his own medical ailments. His story gained attention after he grew over 1500 plants to produce the oil (for free distribution) and subsequently faced significant legal consequences. His efforts spawned a number of other personal documentaries outlining the benefits of cannabis oil in individuals who chose to go public with their stories, and now a large number of these testimonials are available on the internet with written and video accounting of individual's disease progress.

Compelling personal accounts of patients achieving a cure is likely to elicit strong emotions in even the most reluctant reader. Science has demonstrated significant benefits of cannabinoids in multiple disease areas, but accounts of miraculous cures must of course be interpreted with skepticism. Whether the hopes raised by these stories is hype remains to be seen, and patient education is vital in setting reasonable expectations.

Interested adults can now acquire extracts in a variety of manners— including a number of advocate organizations, the internet, or even performing extracts on plants they grow legally at home. Some states allow for the personal controlled cultivation of a limited number of plants, so skilled patients would then even be able to extract cannabinoids from their plants at home. The oil yielded from the extracting process is not precisely predictable in amount or composition, so commercially-available products with labels and safety precautions are preferable for all but experienced home extractors.

For cutting-edge manufacturers, the extraction process can be taken forward to a very sophisticated level. Typically, the raw plant materials are subjected to solvents which dissolve the valuable oils from the plant matter. Solvents can include hydrocarbons such as butane, or alcohols such as ethanol that are suitable to the lipophilic nature of the desired compounds. Rather than a chemical solvent, pressurized carbon dioxide extraction offers the advantage of low residuals and environmental impact; however, it is more technically complex and expensive than other methods.

After removal of the plant solids and any residual solvent, a concentrate remains containing cannabinoids, terpenes and flavonoids. The resulting extract contains a blend of cannabinoid and other compounds based upon the genetics and growing environment of the cultivated plant. This cannabinoids can then be separated from other compounds like the terpenes based on

The temperature at which the extraction and fractionation occurs can affect volatile compounds such as terpenes, so the process by which individual manufacturers process their extracts affects the end product.

Medical Cannabis Dispensary Products

Medical dispensaries vary from state to state with regards to what products can be offered, and in what forms. Some states allow for whole buds, whereas others allow for only extracted forms. State regulations regarding the packaging, labelling, and testing of cannabis-based medicines also varies from state to state. When cannabis was universally an illegal substance, testing for potency and adulterants was not possible, but this is now widely available, and required in some states. Accredited laboratories are now able test samples for the cannabinoid profile and potency as well contaminants such as residual solvents, microbials including fungus, heavy metals, and pesticides.

Unfractionated herbal cannabis:

As previously discussed, there is variability in THC and CBD content in the whole plant based on strain genetics and growing environment. However buds and extracts available in medical dispensaries have the distinct advantage of advertised chemical composition for the major cannabinoids. Below is a depiction of how medical buds might be identified *(for illustrative use only, public domain images)*.

Table 4: Examples of Cannabis Bud Content

Representative photo	Name	Strain	%THC	%CBD
	Example A	Sativa	21.2%	0.3%
	Example B	Sativa	14.7%	14.2%
	Example C	Indica	1.1%	18.5%

There is no ratio of CBD:THC that can be generally described as ideal. For an 8 year-old pediatric epilepsy patient, 20:1 CBD:THC or even higher might be advisable, whereas a 50 year-old anorexic cancer patient may benefit more from a 1:4 ratio. In most cases, evidence does suggest that a balanced approach is best to avoid excess side effects.

Extracts

Due to preference and/or state mandate, some dispensaries offer only extracts. As discussed above, extracting the active ingredients from the flowers and leaves allows for consumption without combustion, as well as more controlled components. With specialized equipment and engineering, extracts can be even further fractionated into cannabinoids and terpenes. This breakdown does allow for customization of ratios outside of the plant's genetics, and also allows the product to become more standardized and consistent with regards to the major cannabinoids. Extracts are often easier to measure than attempting to quantify puffs of a cigarette, so dosing can be more precise with flexible consumption options. On the downside, the approach can counter the entourage effect and possible lost benefits from synergistic effects of the whole herb.

Infusions and Edibles

Whole cannabis or cannabinoids can be solubilized into other lipophilic media such as butters and coconut oil, as well as alcohols. Without overheating beyond 200°C, cannabis-infused oils or butters can be cooked into a variety of edible products that could differ very little from the unmedicated version.

Pharmaceuticals

Dronabinol (Marinol®): a capsule commonly provided in 2.5, 5 and 10 mg dosages. The active ingredient is synthetic trans-isomer THC, suspended in sesame oil. Because of the oral route of administration, the absorption, pharmacokinetics, and metabolism the amount of THC that enters the bloodstream is variable, as discussed below. Currently Schedule III in the United States, it was FDA-approved for use in chemotherapy-induced refractory nausea and vomiting in 1985, and AIDS-related anorexia in 1992.

Nabilone (Casamet®): a synthetic cannabinoid most similar in structure to THC and dronabinol, pictured below. Like dronabinol, it has been approved for refractory chemotherapy-related nausea and vomiting since the 1980's, but was not actively marketed in the United States until 2006. Metabolism and bioavailability mirror THC and dronabinol; however, a significant difference is that the DEA has categorized nabilone as Schedule II.

Nabiximols/Sativex®: comprised of 50% THC and 50% CBD, this is a sublingual spray that has the advantage of avoiding the absorptive and metabolic variability found in oral medications. Because of the shorter duration to active effect, patients are also able to titrate their dose based on a range of sprays per day (Bayer Pharmaceuticals 2014). Developed in Great Britain and studied there since 1999, it has recently received the following recommendation from the All Wales Medicines Strategy Group: Delta-9-tetrahydrocannabinol/ cannabidiol (Sativex®) is recommended as an option for use within NHS Wales as treatment for symptom improvement in adult patients with moderate to severe spasticity due to multiple sclerosis who have not responded adequately to other anti-spasticity medication and who demonstrate clinically significant improvement in spasticity related symptoms during an initial trial of therapy. (All Wales Medicines Strategy Group 2014). It has also been placed in Fast Track status by the US FDA for the treatment of cancer pain.

Cannador®: not available in the United States, this preparation is a capsule of whole plant extracts in a standardized CBD:THC ratio of 1:2, containing approximately 2.5 mg of THC and 1.25 mg of CBD in each capsule. It has been used in smaller studies of MS-related spasticity as well as cancer-related anorexia.

Cannabidol (Epidiolex®): plant-derived CBD. After preliminary studies showed benefit in pediatric epilepsy, it was granted orphan drug status in the United States. GW pharmaceuticals in Great Britain began cultivating high-CBD strains back in 1998, and this particular medication is produced from their crops. It is almost

100% CBD, so has nearly no psychoactive effects which makes it more acceptable for pediatric use.

After the news reports regarding high CBD strains, patients and families may be seeking alternative sources of CBD online. In the US, a strict interpretation of federal guidelines is that any form of marijuana or hemp is illegal. However a quick search of the internet reveals that CBD products are widely available as natural supplements. Without FDA-sanctioned quality or testing guidelines, it may be difficult for patients or physicians to know the exact potency or purity of these products. Preparations currently available commercially on the internet contain doses far lower than the therapeutic doses studied, which would require purchase of relatively large quantities of product.

Table 5: Summary of Common Cannabis-Based Medicine Forms

	Dronabinol	Nabilone	Nabiximols	Cannabidiol	Cannabis
Active ingredient	Synthetic THC	Synthetic THC analog	1:1 plant-based THC/CBD	~99% CBD	Mixture, typically >4% THC
Forms	Capsules	Capsules	Sublingual spray	Liquid, capsules	Inhaled, ingested
Doses	2.5-10 mg peri-chemo	1-2 mg peri-chemo	2.5mg/2.7mg per spray, up to 12 sprays per day	0.5-5 mg/lb/day, or 100-300 mg/d in adults	500 mg herb/cigarette = 20 mg THC, 0.25 mg/kg/d

Table 6: Drug Enforcement Agency (DEA) Schedules of Medications

Schedule	Examples
Schedule I drugs, substances, or chemicals are defined as drugs with no currently accepted medical use and a high potential for abuse. Schedule I drugs are the most dangerous drugs with potentially severe psychological or physical dependence.	heroin, LSD, marijuana (cannabis), ecstasy, and peyote
Schedule II: drugs with a high potential for abuse, less abuse potential than Schedule I drugs, with use potentially leading to severe psychological or physical dependence. These drugs are also considered dangerous.	cocaine, methamphetamine, methadone, hydromorphone, meperidine, oxycodone, fentanyl, Dexedrine, Adderall, and Ritalin
Schedule III: drugs with a moderate to low potential for physical and psychological dependence. Schedule III drugs abuse potential is less than Schedule I and Schedule II drugs but more than Schedule IV.	Codeine, ketamine, anabolic steroids
Schedule IV: drugs with a low potential for abuse and low risk of dependence	Xanax, Soma, Valium, Ativan, Talwin, Ambien
Schedule V: drugs with lower potential for abuse than Schedule IV and consist of preparations containing limited quantities of certain narcotics	Robitussin, Lomotil, Lyrica

Source: http://www.justice.gov/dea/druginfo/ds.shtml

Routes of Systemic Administration

Like endocannabinoids, cannabinoids such as THC and CBD belong to a family of lipophilic fatty acids. The central nervous system is also lipophilic, and cannabinoids can cross the blood-brain barrier. Depending on the route of administration, the cannabinoid will enter the bloodstream and the neurons at different rates.

Inhalation:

Likely the most common route of cannabis intake, since it achieves decarboxylation and absorption very quickly. The main advantage to inhaled methods is a near-immediate absorption of cannabinoids into the bloodstream. Unfortunately, the traditional "smoking" method produces harmful products of combustion such as carbon monoxide found in both tobacco and cannabis smoke. Lacking a filter, smoked marijuana actually has higher levels of tar products such as benz-α-anthracene and benzo-α-pyrene (Wu 1988). Smokers of tobacco and cannabis products alike experience increase pulmonary symptoms such as throat irritation, increased mucus production and bronchitis. Over half of THC is lost to pyrolysis and sidestream smoke with conventional smoking methods, but by avoiding the gastrointestinal tract, more predictable absorption is achieved.

Combustion-based smoking of marijuana products can be associated with a number of pulmonary consequences. Most commonly, users display an increased prevalence of bronchitis-like symptoms. In immunocompromised individuals such as those that are HIV-positive, an increased likelihood of opportunistic infections was also seen. Immunohistochemical staining of the epithelium of chronic marijuana smokers displayed an increased expression of epidermal growth factor receptor, which is a concerning precursor for the development of bronchoalveolar cancer. However, there is been no conclusive evidence that marijuana smoking is associated with an increased risk of cancer (Medicine, Institute of 1999), (Hashibe 2006).

Figure 13: Smoking a Common Marijuana Cigarette (Public domain, WikiCommons)

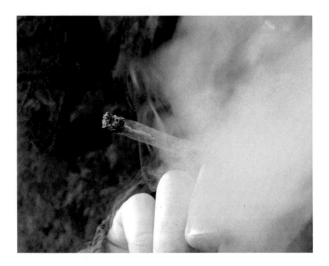

The smoking of any substance will not likely gain favor in the minds of many medical professionals, and in many states that have legislated medical marijuana laws, combustion smoking is not considered a medicinal route. Older studies reported the dangers of marijuana, many of which could be attributed to the smoking itself rather than what substance was smoked. In light of the clinical nature of this

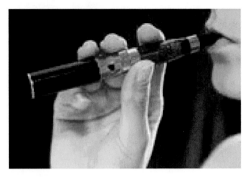

work, information presented will focus on more modern and medically-acceptable routes of cannabinoid intake.

An alternative known as vaporization does heat the product to an inhalable vapor, however combustion does not occur due to lower, controlled heating temperatures.   Generally the oral uptake of cannabinoids is much more variable than inhalation, and will display more erratic blood levels due to variability in absorption and metabolism. Vaporization through a variety of commercially-available devices, including a heating device with a vapor collection bag, as well as smaller electronic "cigarettes", has been shown to be an effective delivery route for inhaled cannabis and cannabis extracts (D. Abrams 2007).

The vaporization of cannabis products offers a number of advantages over both the oral route and traditional smoking: (Gieringer 2004)

- avoiding carcinogenic hydrocarbons and carbon monoxide combustion byproducts
- preservation of near-immediate absorption and symptom relief

- ability to titrate dosing based on the short-acting effects and ability to re-dose

The lower temperature produced in vaporizers likely also preserves the activity of more terpenes, which become a vapor at around the same boiling point as THC. A temperature of approximately 185°C (365°F) will vaporize the majority of THC. Other more harmful vapors appeared over 200°C, with true combustion around 220-230°C.

Vaporization is not entirely harmless. Like electronic tobacco cigarettes, the active ingredient is accompanied by other chemicals required for extraction and suspension. Close inspection of the ingredients is warranted to avoid exposure to excess propylene glycol or other residual solvents.

Oral/per os (PO):

This refers to the most common overall route of medication administration, which is swallowing a capsule or pill. The medication is absorbed through the gastrointestinal tract, and metabolized by the liver. THC undergoes degradation by stomach acid, so meal intake and stomach acidity are additional variables affecting oral THC absorption. Onset occurs in about 30min to 2h, but duration can be as long as 8-10 hours. As discussed in the pharmacology section, the first-pass metabolite 11-OH THC is psychoactive, which may enhance and lengthen the subjective effects. For edible products such as brownies or cookies, the total

THC content in milligrams as well as the serving size must be read carefully to avoid accidental overconsumption.

Due to the very long time of onset (up to 3 hours) with many ingested forms of cannabis, there is significantly more difficulty with dose titration and an increased likelihood of premature re-dosing with subsequent over-medication. This risk is most likely with new users, such as many cannabis-naïve patients that may be enrolling in new state medical cannabis programs or visiting states with recreational marijuana legislation.

Urban folklore has long relayed tales of persons accidentally eating marijuana brownies. In 2007, a Michigan police officer ingested marijuana brownies that he confiscated from a suspect, but his lack of experience with ingesting THC led him and his wife to call 911 fearful of a lethal overdose. The incident was broadcast on the news, along with the recording of his 911 call. Recently a prominent New York Times author wrote about her experience underestimating the effects of edible marijuana products while sampling recreational products in Colorado, which highlights how simple it might be to over-ingest THC in the edible preparations that are widely available today (Dowd 2014).

Transmucosal:

Cannabinoid preparations can be administered via various mucous membranes, most commonly sublingually or buccal, as well as intranasal or rectal. Even ocular drops can be manufactured by using newer technology to make the cannabinoids more soluble in water.

By avoiding first pass metabolism through the liver, bioavailability via mucosal absorption is more consistent than oral. Another advantage is the avoidance of smoking or vaporization of any kind, which minimizes secondhand exposure.

For rectal suppositories, THC is chemically modified to the hemisuccinate, but has demonstrated roughly twice the bioavailability of the oral route in limited studies. This route also offers advantages to treat disease states in which the oral route may be unsafe such as seizure disorders or aspiration risk (F. e. Grotenhermen 2002).

Transdermal:
In this case a medication is absorbed directly through the skin, through the use of a patch or ointment. This route does offer the advantages of a more constant level of medication delivery, however absorption of medication through the various layers of the skin can be more variable, and additional variability regarding adhesive and other inactive supportive chemicals can make this method less desirable.

Due to effects upon the TRPV1 receptor that are similar to capsaicin, cannabinoids have potential as pain-relieving patches. Patches containing a variety of cannabinoids are currently commercially available in medical cannabis states, including THC, CBD, 1:1 THC to CBD, and CBN.

Cautions

Unlike the vast majority of chemicals used for medical treatment, isolated cannabis has never been definitively shown to produce lethal effects in humans. Survey data indicating the widespread use of cannabis in the US and other countries is also reassuring regarding the volume and duration of cannabis use in millions of persons without report of lethality. Taken together, data would indicate that cannabis has a favorable safety profile both in laboratory animals and in everyday human use.

However, any chemical with active effects upon human chemistry must be used with thoughtfulness. A licensed provider recommending medical cannabis should do so with knowledge of pharmacology and attention to each individual patient's underlying medical state—the same caution required with any other medication. Because therapeutic cannabis is a newly developing field, additional educational resources may be needed to bring both patients and medical prescribers up to speed with the state of cannabis research and practical use. In the end, the professional judgment of the licensed medical provider will determine the potential risks and benefits of cannabis use for each individual patient before making a recommendation.

Underlying disease processes

Cardiovascular Disease:

THC has effects upon the cardiovascular system through multiple sites of action. Initially, vasodilation and reflex tachycardia may be observed, but chronic use of THC can lead to less predictable outcomes. The exact effect of cannabinoids on the sympathetic and parasympathetic systems, baroreceptors, and vascular endothelium is yet to be fully determined, and could be influenced by the common practice of breath-holding during cannabis inhalation. A growing number of case reports have highlighted the cardiovascular risks with regard to angina, acute coronary events, cerebrovascular events, and arrhythmias (Thomas 2014); however, it is difficult to interpret which risks are attributable to cannabinoids themselves versus the effects of smoking and concurrent tobacco use. Research into the mechanism of these cardiovascular events found that the cause could be related to platelet activation. CB1 and CB2 receptors are both found on human platelet cells, however the mechanism appears to be related to the arachidonic acid that is produced by enzymatic breakdown of endogenous and exogenous cannabinoids (Brantl 2014).

Overall, this evidence may lead a provider to exercise caution recommending THC-containing compounds to individuals prone to cardiovascular morbidity.

Pulmonary Disease:

Not surprisingly, users of smoked marijuana cigarettes experience increased rates of bronchitis-like symptoms such as cough and sputum. There is no evidence of increased emphysema in cannabis-only smokers, and no clear evidence for increased cancer risk in case-control studies (Aldingtoon 2008). A large cohort of 64,855 Kaiser Permanante patients found no increase in respiratory cancers either. Regardless, smoking any substance is not advisable for persons with pulmonary disease and other routes of cannabis intake are available.

Interactions

Cannabinoids are highly protein-bound due to hydrophobic structure, which could potentiate interaction with other highly protein-bound medications. At this time, displacement of protein-bound medications by cannabinoids has not been demonstrated in humans so this may not be clinically significant.

In modern medicine where polypharmacy is common, interactions at the P450 system may be of clinical relevance. Cannabinoids are metabolized by the P450 system, and as competitors for metabolism, drug levels of some common medications may be affected. CBD is typically quite benign, but as a potent p450 inhibitor, patients on certain medications will require extra caution if they are on large doses of CBD.

Table 7: Common medications metabolized by the p450 system

2C9	3A4
Ibuprofen, naproxen	Erythromycin
Glipizide	Quinidine
Losartan	Benzodiazepines
Amitriptyline	cyclosporine
Fluoxetine	Calcium channel blockers
phenytoin	lovastatin
warfarin	Estrogen, testosterone
	Cocaine, codeine, methadone

Polypharmacy

In addition to the interactions noted above at a molecular level, at the organism level, the additive effects of other sedative medications should also be considered. Mixing medications for anxiety, sleep and pain with medical cannabis could lead to oversedation.

Previous studies have demonstrated that patient understanding of prescription labels is limited by patient literacy rates and the number of prescriptions they must maintain (Davis 2006). Chronically ill patients seeking relief from cannabis are likely taking other prescriptions, some of which may have additive mind-altering effects that further impair their ability to track multiple medications. Taking additional time to educate patients and reinforce medication instructions in a fashion fitting to the patient is required to avoid misunderstanding and noncompliance.

Driving

Cannabis is known to be associated with functional impairment on multiple neurocognitive measures that correlate with driving: attention, vigilance, tracking, time perception, and motor coordination. However the amount of cannabis required to cause significant impairment varies by the user's metabolism, experience with cannabis, and experience with driving. Furthermore, laboratory neurocognitive studies do not directly translate into real-world driving tests, where experienced cannabis users often show little functional impairment (Sewell 2009).

The effect of cannabinoids with regards to driving impairment is difficult to quantify. Unlike the hydrophilic alcohol, where the dose and route of administration is more easily quantifiable, cannabinoids are ingested in a variety of forms and display variable absorption and metabolism. There is no national standardized plasma concentration at which an individual could be considered too impaired to participate in activities such as driving or legal matters, but the state of Colorado is using 5 ng/mL as the basis of new driving under the influence legislation (Colorado Department of Transportation 2014), and Washington state may follow. This is correlated to multiple studies evaluating both culpability for motor vehicle fatalities and driving under the influence arrests, where an odds ratio (OR) was calculated for THC-positive drivers versus drug-free drivers. An OR at 5 ng/mL for THC was found to exceed the OR for a blood alcohol concentration of 0.1-0.15% (Drummer 2004), which suggests similar levels of driving impairment at these two levels. Previous studies that did not clarify the blood level, using only positive or negative, were unable to show that cannabis was associated with driving injuries, with an OR slightly less than 1.

Other countries have legislation regarding blood levels lower than 5 ng/mL, such as 2.2 in Sweden, and zero-tolerance in Australia (Hartmann 2013). Due to the erratic absorption and metabolism, retroactively determining the blood level at the time of the driving infraction versus the time of the blood draw cannot be done reliably.

Drivers <25 years old account for a disproportionate number of traffic fatalities. This younger group of drivers is also more prone to risk-taking behaviors such as alcohol and drug misuse, risk-taking behaviors, and overconfidence. Lacking the driving skills acquired over years of experience, younger drivers may suffer more driving impairment while under the influence of cannabis and/or alcohol, and particularly while under the influence of both.

The National Highway Traffic Safety Administration Drug and Human Performance Fact Sheet for cannabis indicates that driving performance is impaired for approximately three hours, including decreased car handling performance, decreased reaction time, impaired time and distance estimation, motor incoordination, and sleepiness, but also stipulates that it is impossible to predict specific effects based on blood THC or THC-COOH concentrations (National Highway Traffic Safety Administration n.d.).

Regardless of the numeric levels of intoxicant, field sobriety test have been designed to assess the level of substance-induced impairment. In a standard field sobriety test, a number of maneuvers are used to assess the motor coordination of the driver, including nystagmus, walk-and-turn, and one-leg stand. In many cases, an individual intoxicated on THC would fail roadside sobriety testing. Many states such as Colorado have begun specific training for drug intoxication recognition.

Youth

The endocannabinoid system is widespread throughout the CNS, and develops with the brain throughout childhood and adolescence. Introducing chemicals such as cannabis, psychotropics, amphetamines, and other psychoactive chemicals affects neural activity in the developing brain.

A number of studies have shown that persons who choose to use cannabis in the teenage years displayed long-term effects such loss of cognition and behavioral problems (Gonzalez 2012). One study in New Zealand found an 8-point reduction in IQ in heavy teenage smokers, and more importantly, the cognitive and behavioral problems are not regained. In the case of youth cannabis use, it is difficult to determine the causality of these harmful effects. In the case of a troubled youth who is using illegal marijuana, there are likely associated familial and societal confounders contributing to the long-term difficulties reported in this population. In persons who began smoking cannabis as a youth, reduced activity in prefrontal regions and hippocampus can be seen, which reinforces the effects upon developing brain matter (Volkow 2014).

In the War on Drugs, cannabis was portrayed as a gateway drug for youth. This has not been a persistent concept, but because cannabis does have effects on the reward center of the brain, it could indeed alter reward center development if used before brain maturation. Conversely, in adult users of cannabis, it can act as a substitute for "harder" drugs including alcohol.

Figure 14: Percentage of 12th graders reporting a substance is fairly easy or very easy to get

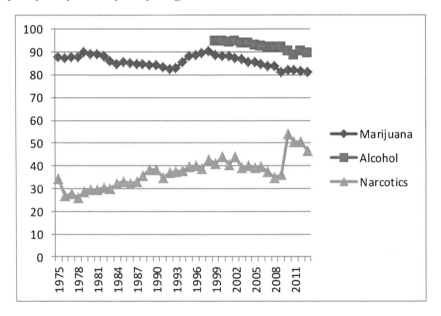

Source: The Monitoring the Future Study, the University of Michigan, http://www.monitoringthefuture.org/data/13data/13drtbl14.pdf. In 2010, the question regarding narcotics was changed to include Vicodin, Percocet, Oxycontin

With more and more states decriminalizing and/or supporting the medical use of cannabis, a valid concern is raised that impressionable youth may mistakenly believe that all cannabis use is

"OK", and increased rates of adolescent marijuana use will result. Indeed, a parallel could be drawn between cannabis products and the widespread societal acceptance of mind-altering prescriptions such as sleeping pills and pain pills. Complex family and social dynamics is outside the scope of this work, but the information presented here would certainly indicate that recreational marijuana use amongst underage persons is not acceptable. Accurate education of parents and the community, as well as open and honest communication with medical providers, will dispel myths and promote responsible parenting practices.

All cannabis products should be properly labelled, kept in child-proof containers, and stored in a fashion that avoids accidental ingestion by children or impaired adults. While stories about accidental ingestion of "pot brownies" can a humorous component of urban lore, this can represent a real danger for the psyche of children. With the development of multiple edible products in states such as Colorado, it is easy to see how candies and brownies could lead to accidental ingestion if these products are not labelled and stored safely.

Pregnancy/Lactation

THC and its metabolites have been shown to cross the placenta and into breast milk. Due to its effects on nausea, cannabis may be sought by pregnant women suffering from morning sickness or hyperemesis gravidarum, but there are no studies to support the safe use of cannabis in pregnancy or breast feeding. Dronabinol, synthetic THC, is pregnancy category C, which indicates limited teratogenicity studies in rats have not revealed overt dangers, but there no adequate studies in pregnant humans.

Pregnant mothers who smoke cannabis or other combustibles inhale increased carbon monoxide, which deprives the fetus of oxygen, a known harm to the fetus. As with studies on youth, alteration of developing brain chemistry with exogenous neuromodulators could have long-term effects. A 2013 review article in *Pediatrics* outlined effects of prenatal THC exposure, and in summary found no evidence for physical malformations, but mixed evidence for fetal growth, withdrawal irritability, and long-term cognitive linguistic and behavioral measures (M. a. Behnke 2013).

Studies examining prenatal exposure to cannabis and the long-term effects on the neonate should be interpreted with an eye for confounders rather than causality. For instance, one study found that maternal use of THC during the 2nd and 3rd trimester predicted depressive symptoms 10 years later in the offspring (Gray 2005). If further questioning determined that the mother was using THC for her own depression, then both the genetic and environmental effects of maternal depression would influence depression incidence in her children. Additionally, maternal use of an illicit substance would imply an element of substance addiction, would also has heritability.

To date, there are no published studies regarding CBD-only formulations.

Psychiatry

Conventional wisdom is to avoid cannabis in persons at high risk for psychiatric disease. This recommendation is again based upon older studies in which cannabis containing primarily THC, with only traces of other cannabinoids, was found to be associated with a higher risk of psychotic symptoms and/or diagnoses. A foundational Swedish questionnaire study followed a large cohort of 45,570 military enrollees and found a dose-dependent relative risk of schizophrenia of 3 for conscripts who had used cannabis between 1-50 times, and 6 for conscripts who had used cannabis >50 times over 15 years (Andreasson 1987).

Epidemiologic studies along this line did continue, and continued to associate cannabis use with schizophrenia and/or psychosis at a relative risk of approximately 2 for adult cannabis initiation, and higher for those who began as a youth. In addition to this association, some studies found that in patients with psychotic prodromal symptomatology, that cannabis use could provoke full-blown symptoms (van der Meer 2012). Drawing a causal relationship is still not solidified, since persons with mental health disorders often self-medicate with cannabis and other mind-altering substances (W. e. Hall 2004) and the underlying etiology of schizophrenia remains elusive. Studies evaluating the etiology of schizophrenia have identified a genetic predisposition at COMT, CNR1, BDNF, AKT1 and NRG1 that may cause a person to be more susceptible to the psychic stress of cannabis use (Pelayo-Teran 2012). Also, as emphasized in other areas, a higher CBD content prevents unpleasant psychic experiences (Schubart 2011), and CBD is a growing area for treatment of mental disorders such as schizophrenia.

Addiction/Abuse

In the context of a federally illegal substance such as cannabis, questions regarding the potential for abuse and addiction are apt to arise. Like anxiety and pain medications, providers should exercise caution in recommending any mind-altering substance to a patient with a history of addiction or high potential for such.

2012 National Survey on Drug Abuse and Health, 8.6 million Americans meet criteria for alcohol, 5.1 million for any drug, and 2.7 for marijuana (Center for Behavioral Health Statistics and Quality 2013). The high baseline prevalence of substance-related disorders in potential medical cannabis patients may influence a provider to screen for addictive behaviors with a tool such as SBIRT (Screening, Brief Intervention, and Referral to Treatment) before recommending a psychoactive substance such as cannabis, or prescribing psychoactive substances such as opiates or amphetamine derivatives.

In the case of substance abuse, addiction can be broadly described as a person continuing to use the substance even though it has led to negative life consequences. The National Institute on Drug Abuse (NIDA) estimates that 9% of adults who use cannabis will display elements of addiction, but the number rises to 17% in those that began using marijuana between ages 13-25. Compared to other substances, cannabis does have a lower lifetime risk of dependence: (Anthony 1994)

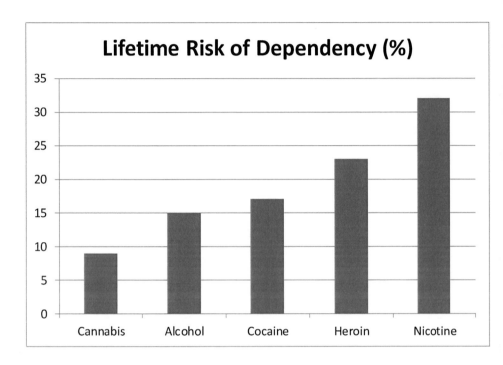

A withdrawal syndrome has now been recognized in the American Psychiatric Association (APA) DSM-V including anxiety, irritability and sleep disruption (Budney 2004), and would be characterized as mild in comparison to withdrawal from other substances such as alcohol or opiates, but more similar to nicotine or caffeine. This is most commonly seen in chronic daily users who cease abruptly. The APA's Charles O'Brien, MD, PhD also clarified their stance on addiction versus dependence:

The term dependence is misleading, because people confuse it with addiction, when in fact the tolerance and withdrawal patients experience are very normal responses to prescribed medications that affect the central nervous system. On the other hand, addiction is compulsive drug-seeking behavior which is quite different. We hope that this new classification will help end this wide-spread misunderstanding.

Review of Cannabinoid Treatment for Selected disorders

Background

While a body of research exists regarding treatment for a number of conditions, review of the literature must be undertaken with an understanding of the cannabis compounds used at the time. Early research involved undifferentiated cannabis, which would likely be best translated into current treatment modalities using whole dried smoked marijuana plant material. In particular, FDA-endorsed research within the United States is limited to cannabis regulated by the National Institute on Drug Abuse (NIDA) and grown at the University of Mississippi by contract. Historically distributed strains of marijuana plant matter contained about 3.5-4% THC and no CBD, so research findings should be interpreted within this context. Now, the Mississippi facility has expanded the range of THC available, such as low (2%), medium (4%) and high (8%), and is reported to stock strains up to 14%. Health Canada currently distributes marijuana dried leaves at about 11-15% THC (Health Canada 2007).

Even NIDA has had to respond to the increased need for suitable cannabis supplies for research purposes. In late August 2014, they requested a massive increase in their quota for cannabis production through the University of Mississippi-- from 21 kg to 650 kg (Drug

Enforcement Agency 2014). In particular, the increased demand for high-CBD strains and the state specific legislation that has passed in 2014 to support the demand will require dramatically different approach toward the cultivation of cannabis products for federally-approved research. Due to the time required to grow the plants to maturity, this increased supply will have some delay before it is available.

With an understanding of the endocannabinoid functions, it is not surprising that exogenous cannabinoids can have widespread effects upon the nervous system. While cannabis is still used for its long-standing indications of nausea, anorexia, and glaucoma, further study of the endocannabinoid system, its receptors, its natural and synthetic ligands are taking the field of medical cannabis research in new directions. One new area of study is neuroprotection from the neurotoxic effects of hyperexcitability, free radical damage and ultimately cellular apoptosis. In this process, a cellular insult such as hypoxia or hypoglycemia leads to a variety of downstream effects. This includes an excess production of excitatory neurotransmitter such as glutamate, which in turn results in increased NMDA receptor sensitivity and excess calcium influx. Nitric oxide production also synergizes apoptosis, and results in oxidative free radical production. These free radicals lead to further damage, which perpetuates this neurotoxic process. CBD can temper this process through its effects as antioxidant free radical scavenger, as well as modulation of calcium influx.

Another new area of cannabis-based treatment involves the immune system. CB2 receptors are found in CNS microglia, along with CB1 receptors at lower levels. CBD and CB2 receptor agonists are able to quell inflammation in the delicate neural tissues, and potentially offer benefit in neuroinflammatory and neurodegenerative disorders.

Review of Specific Medical Conditions

Seizure disorders

Previous studies reported concern that seizure frequency may be increased in marijuana smokers. At that time, this would have described smokers of traditional marijuana cigarettes, which is a far cry from how cannabis is being used with regard to epilepsy today.

Seizure disorders affect approximately three million Americans, more patients than any of the other conditions commonly treated by cannabinoids. Studies regarding epilepsy and cannabis began long ago, in the Mechoulam laboratory (Carlini 1975) and expanded exponentially upon the elucidation of cannabis constituents and their varying mechanisms of action.

THC, acting as an agonist at cannabinoid receptors, may still have a mixed excitatory/inhibitory effect upon brain systems involved in epilepsy due to the opposing neurotransmitters involved in anatomic pathways, which likely explains why the reports of THC's epileptic effects are mixed (R. Pertwee 2008). In contrast, CBD has inhibitory effects at cannabinoid receptors CB1, CB2 and GPR55, and in vivo its general effect upon hyperexcitable neural tissues appears to be inhibitory as well, which makes it a good candidate for antiepileptic treatment.

More recently, the use of CBD in particular for the treatment of seizure disorders was brought to the forefront by Dr. Sanjay Gupta (CNN 2013). In a televised special called Weed, Dr. Gupta chose to recant his previous opinions regarding cannabis, and promote the use of high-CBD cannabis in the treatment of Charlotte Figi's refractory Dravet epilepsy syndrome. The strain of high-CBD cannabis used was developed in Colorado, and there is now a long waiting list of patients hoping to gain benefit.

The recent publicity powered a wave of grass-roots pressure on state legislatures, which has already resulted in a number states passing legislation that considers therapeutic hemp separately from marijuana. The lack of psychoactivity in CBD-only products makes these products far less controversial than cannabis initiatives in general. In July 2014, H.R. 5226 was presented to Congress, entitled "Charlotte's Web Medical Hemp Act of 2014" (Perry 2014). The passage of this bill would provide federal uniformity in tolerance for CBD and hemp products instead of patchwork state regulations. To be considered a hemp product, the cannabis sativa plant materials, alive or not, must contain <0.3% THC by dry weight.

GW Pharmaceuticals has a high-CBD product as well, Epidiolex®, that is derived from plants grown in the UK. The company has received both orphan drug designation and Fast Track designation from the FDA for this CBD-only medication. Expanded access studies are underway for refractory pediatric epilepsy in California and New York, and the company just released preliminary results on 27 patients who had completed 12 weeks of adjunctive Sativex®

therapy, with response quantified by % change in seizure frequency average over four weeks, as compared to baseline. The overall reduction in seizure frequency was 44%, and 15% were seizure-free. In the Dravet subset (n=9), the mean reduction in seizure frequency was 52%, with 33% achieving seizure-free status. Most patients did experience at least one side effects, including somnolence, fatigue, diarrhea, and appetite changes. Three patients are being withdrawn due to lack of effect.

Multiple sclerosis (MS)

MS is the most common inflammatory disease of the central nervous system. The incidence of MS varies depending on the population and geographic area, but ranges from less than 5 to 200 per 100,000 persons (Mayr WT n.d.) Spasticity is a common and debilitating symptom, which affects daily life in about one-third of MS patients (Rizzo MA 2004).

In Europe, cannabis has been explored as a treatment option for MS for many years. As early as 1997, a survey reported improved pain and spasticity with cannabis use (Consroe 1997) and subsequent trials seemed to support the beneficial effect (Petro & Ellenberger). Fortunately their years of experience using cannabinoids and the clinical studies they have published have solidified the therapeutic uses and safety profile.

Because the endocannabinoid system is distributed throughout the CNS, broad cannabinoid treatment in MS affect the motor control areas, pain perception areas, as well as the glial cells that mediate autoimmune inflammation (D. a. Baker 2008). Randomized controlled trials such as CUPID evaluated dronabinol alone in disease progression, which did not show benefit (Zajicek 2013), but did not incorporate the anti-inflammatory effects of CBD.

Sativex, a combination of 1:1 THC:CBD is a sublingual spray approved for use in Europe for the treatment of pain and spasticity in

MS patients. In the United States, the combination medication is under investigational use in phase III clinical trials, and has granted Fast Track status for approval in treatment of cancer pain. Initial benefits in spasticity were shown to be prolonged long-term as monitoring continued in the MOVE trial, without reports of serious adverse events (Flachenecker 2014). Treatment tolerance was also documented in long-term follow-up in the UK (Serpell 2013), with adverse effects including dizziness (24.7%) and fatigue (12.3%).

Figure 14: MRI of MS lesions

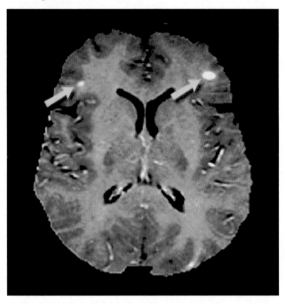

In addition to the known effects upon spasticity, a neuromodulatory benefit of cannabis may benefit as well. MS patients often have monoclonal antibodies as evidence of the underlying autoimmune response to myelin basic protein. Current disease-modifying therapies in MS are designed to modify this immune response, by reducing the TH1 response, by increasing TH2 response, and by limiting T cell migration into the CNS. Pathologic evidence suggests that apoptosis, perhaps triggered by excitotoxicity, may be the primary event preceding inflammation and lesion formation in patients with relapsing-remitting MS (Matute 2001).

Amyotrophic Lateral Sclerosis (ALS)

In some ways similar to MS, ALS is characterized by motor neuron degeneration and death with gliosis replacing lost neurons. In some familial cases, mutations in superoxide dismutase (SOD1) trigger superoxide radicals, setting off an inflammatory cascade which activates microglial cells. Once activated, microglial cells perpetuate the pathologic inflammatory responses by releasing additional oxygen radicals, excess excitatory glutamate, and cytokines that promote further immune cell migration into the CNS. Activated microglia behave much like activated macrophages in the periphery, but in the neural tissues the inflammation in ALS can lead to long-term tissue damage and neural degeneration/death. Excess glutamate-mediated excitotoxicity is central to ALS pathophysiology, possibly due to dysfunctional glutamate receptors, so an inhibitory cannabinoid could be of therapeutic value.

In animal models of ALS, a synthetic CB2 receptor agonist was shown to achieve delay in disease progression (Kim 2006). THC has been previously shown to induce a shift from TH1 to TH2 cytokine profiles in T cells, which would modulate immune response favorably in ALS (Wolf 2008).

Aside from disease modification, symptom control in this terminally ill population is vital. Cannabis has been used to treat a number of the symptoms ALS patients suffer, such as spasticity, pain, and nausea (Carter 2001). Antioxidants are a mainstay of therapy, so

CBD and other cannabinoids could achieve the goals of symptom control and disease control simultaneously. ALS patients did report that marijuana relieved major symptoms of their disease except for speech and swallowing difficulties, but access to cannabis treatment is not always available (Amtmann 2004).

Human Immunodeficiency Virus/Acquired Immune Deficiency Syndrome

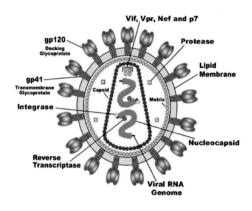

Already used by a significant proportion of patients living with HIV/AIDS (Woolridge 2005), cannabis may help to ameliorate the chronic symptoms of anorexia, nausea, and pain. (Sidney 2001) but conclusive evidence is lacking (Lutge EE 2013).

In more recent years, delineation of the effects of cannabinoids on neurodegenerative disorders shed light upon possible treatment for HIV-Associated Neurocognitive Disorder (HAND). Similarly to other CNS disorders, glial activation is suppressed by CBD and can reduce long-term inflammatory damage. Further inflammatory suppression through CB2-specific treatment would also offer promising benefit (Purohit 2014).

HIV-sensory neuropathy may also benefit from cannabinoid treatment, as was suggested by Dr. Abrams' study of cannabis in painful sensory neuropathy (D. e. Abrams 2007).

Previously, questions about the interactions of cannabinoids and protease inhibitors arose due to the shared hepatic metabolism. Results of this investigation revealed that cannabis produced no significant reduction in protease inhibitor function (Kosel BW 2002), and the use of marijuana is theorized to indirectly improve antiretroviral function by reducing gastrointestinal symptoms and thereby increasing compliance.

Terminal Illness and Palliative Care

Increasing numbers of Americans are choosing hospice for end-of-life care (Thompson 2011). When hospice care was established in the 1970s, cancer patients made up the largest percentage of hospice admissions. Today, cancer diagnoses account for less than half of all hospice admissions (37.7%), with increasing numbers of unspecified debility (13.9%), dementia (12.5%), heart disease (11.4%), and lung disease (8.5%). ALS and AIDS together make up less than 1% (National Hospice and Palliative Care Organization 2012). Despite increasing numbers, palliative care has not enjoyed an insurgence of cannabis-based research, but as more and more patients choose to die at home, that the use of cannabis products to promote end-of-life comfort will increase.

Pain control

In states with well-established registry programs such as AZ, pain is the single most common indication for medical marijuana. However, pain can be a vague term for a number of diagnoses and syndromes that may have differing pathophysiology. Pain caused by a broken bone cannot be compared to pain caused by a phantom limb, by diabetic neuropathy, or metastatic cancer. Similarly, it is difficult to compare human pain perception with pain models in animal research, which uses tests such as tail-flick, paw pressure, and hot plates.

When used appropriately, cannabinoids appear to have great potential in treating particular types of pain. Secondary to the anti-inflammatory effects, rheumatoid arthritis would be an inflammatory condition well-suited to cannabis therapy. Cannabinoids offer anti-inflammatory effect, but through different mechanism than COX, so carry reduced risks for gastrointestinal complications.

Pain perception is a complex process, originating at a site of injury or inflammation, carried through peripheral nerves to the spinal cord "gating" process, then ascending the spinothalamic tract and dorsal column into various areas such as the thalamus, cortex, and periaqueductal gray matter. Because of the multiple synapses involved along this route, the pathway is amenable to therapeutic targets. Leveraging cannabinoids and the TRPV1 receptor may prove to elucidate new ways of treating chronic pain and neuropathic pain, neither of which finding a niche in conventional medical treatments.

The endocannabinoid pathways have even shed new light on acetaminophen, an extremely common medication. After endocannabinoids are cleaved and arachidonic acid is formed by FAAH, acetaminophen combines with arachidonic acid to form a molecule called AM404. AM404 has effects at the TRPV1 receptor, as well as weak agonist effects at cannabinoid receptors, which may mediate acetaminophen's pain-relieving effects (Hogestatt 2005). This finding again demonstrates that the endocannabinoids and their root fatty acids have many areas of interdependency.

Nausea and Vomiting

Controlling nausea and vomiting has been one of the more familiar indications for cannabis-based medicines, supported by the FDA approval of dronabinol for chemotherapy-induced nausea and vomiting in 1985. Later, the FDA rescheduled dronabinol from schedule II to schedule III, indicating a known therapeutic use and a lower potential for addiction. Demonstration of CB1 receptors in the rat area postrema, the "vomiting" center of the brain, supports an objective mechanism for THC mediated symptom control. Additionally, studies have now demonstrated CB receptors in the GI tract, so cannabinoids act upon nausea and vomiting both centrally and peripherally.

A systemic review of cannabinoids for the control of chemotherapy-induced nausea and vomiting showed that cannabis was more effective than conventional antiemetics such as prochlorpromazine and metoclopramide, but also had higher incidence of side effects such as feeling "high", drowsy, dizzy, and either euphoric or dysphoric (Tramer 2001). However, a head-to-head study between isolated cannabis products and newer antiemetics such as odansetron has not been undertaken.

Appetite Stimulation

While suppression of nausea and vomiting can indirectly promote appetite, there is evidence that THC and the CB1 receptor have a more direct role in stimulating appetite

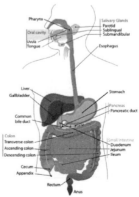

through central pathways. Long known to be a side effect of cannabis, this side effect can be leveraged to benefit patients suffering anorexia and wasting.

In comparison to other agents such as megestrol, a clear benefit has not been shown for cancer-associated anorexia (Jatoi 2002).

Trials in AIDS patients did show benefit versus placebo both short- and long-term regarding appetite stimulation, but less effect upon measured weight gain (Beal 1997).

Inflammatory bowel disease

Inflammatory bowel diseases such as Crohn's and ulcerative colitis stand to benefit from the known anti-inflammatory effects of CBD

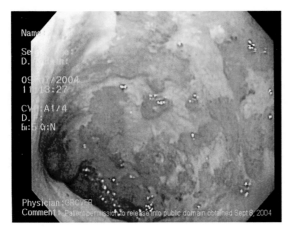

and CB2 agonists together with the antidiarrheal and antiemetic qualities of THC. The gastrointestinal tract has a large volume of nervous tissue, and both CB1 and CB2 are expressed in the mammalian gut (Massa 2005). CBD was shown to reduce colon injury in a murine model of colitis by reducing reactive oxygen species in 2009 (Borelli 2009), and other studies showed that intestinal disease activity correlated with AEA levels in ulcerative colitis and celiac sprue, suggesting again that endocannabinoid manipulation may be of benefit. The first human evaluation came in 2011 with Dr. Naftali's observational study of THC cigarettes in Israel (Naftali, Treatment of Crohn's disease with cannabis: an observational study 2011). A small group of Crohn's disease patients improved clinical scores with the use of cannabis, and could reduce other medications. A followup placebo-controlled study also showed benefit in clinical response (Naftali 2013). Given the short duration of investigation in this field, it is too early to draw conclusions but the underlying principles and initial studies are encouraging.

Glaucoma

Confirmatory to popular lore, studies in the early 1970s showed that marijuana, when smoked, lowered intraocular pressure (IOP) in people with normal pressure and those with glaucoma. In an effort to determine whether marijuana, or drugs derived from marijuana, might be effective as a glaucoma treatment, the National Eye Institute (NEI) supported research studies beginning in 1978. These studies demonstrated that some derivatives of marijuana transiently lowered IOP when administered orally, intravenously, or by smoking, but not when topically applied to the eye. This duration of action was deemed too short to make smoked THC a practical route of delivery for 24-hour intraocular pressure control (National Eye Institute, National Institutes of Health 1997).

However, none of these studies demonstrated that marijuana -- or any of its components -- could lower IOP as effectively as drugs already on the market. In addition, some potentially serious side effects were noted, including an increased heart rate and a decrease in blood pressure in studies using smoked marijuana.

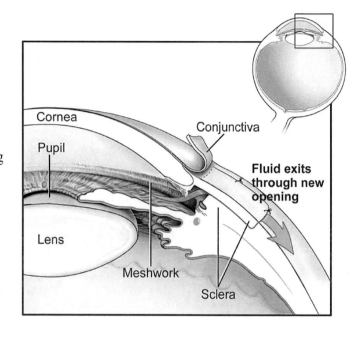

The most recent recommendation from the American Academy of Ophthalmology found "no evidence demonstrating increased benefit and/or diminished risk of marijuana use in the treatment of glaucoma compared with the wide variety of pharmaceutical agents now available." (AAO Complementary Therapy Task Force 2014)

Unfortunately much of the research done in this area was done prior to the advances in molecular biology that identified CB1 mRNA and proteins in the human eye (A. e. Porcella 2000). The synthetic cannabinoid WIN 55212–2 applied topically was shown to reduce intraocular pressure in glaucoma cases resistant to conventional therapies (A. e. Porcella 2001). Recent research with regards to the anti-inflammatory and neuroprotective effects of cannabinoids may lead to advances in the cannabinoid treatment of retinal disorders (Yazulla 2008). Since vision loss in glaucoma is mediated through optic nerve damage, neuroprotective agents would still offer benefit in preventing vision loss in glaucoma and other ophthalmologic disorders.

Because of the lipophilic nature of cannabinoids, an effective aqueous delivery system for ophthalmologic use was difficult to develop. Hydrophobic drug delivery vehicles using cyclodextrins developed in the late 1990s (Jarvinen 2002) which enabled the hydrophobic cannabinoids such as THC and AEA to be soluble in an ophthalmologic preparation. Future research regarding the ophthalmologic benefits of cannabinoids will benefit both from more specific THC doses and from more consistent delivery vehicles.

Tourette's and neurologic tics

Tourette's syndrome is a developmental neuropsychiatric disorder characterized by chronic motor and verbal tics, beginning before age 18. According to the CDC, GTS affects about 2-3/1,000 children aged 6-17. Going back to the 1980s, anecdotal reports began appearing in the literature related to THC use and Gilles de la Tourette syndrome (GTS). Benefits were reported, however the sample sizes were small and the benefits are based upon subjective patient reports. Later, Müller-Vahl published two studies reporting reduction in frequency and severity of tics, but again only a small number of patients (28) participated. Her research, based in Germany, demonstrated some beneficial effects at low doses of THC, titrated upward slowly (Mueller-Vahl 2003).

In review, only these two studies have been conducted and the sample size was not large enough to make any determinations about supporting the use of cannabinoids in treating tics or obsessive behaviors in Tourette's syndrome (Curtis 2009).

Brief Review of Newly Developing Research

Cancer

Reports of the antineoplastic properties of cannabinoids have recently sparked a great deal of excitement regarding the future of cannabis science. Experimental cell cultures of varying cell lines have been treated with CBD and other cannabinoids, and antineoplastic properties such as reduced invasion and reduced proliferation have been seen.

- AEA inhibits breast cancer cell proliferation (Petrocellis 1998)
- CBD, CBG and CBC inhibit breast carcinoma cell growth (Ligestri 2006)
- CBD inhibition of tumor pathways in glial cells (Solinas 2013)
- CBD and high-CBD strain cannabis inhibition of colon carcinogenesis (Romano 2014)

This burgeoning field will likely take some time to clarify, since the mechanism of cannabinoid effect differs by tissue, and different cell lines express different receptors. One example would be antineoplastic effects through the PPAR receptor. Because PPAR is primarily expressed peripherally in adipocytes, cancer cells lines such as liposarcomas and mammary adenocarcinomas often express PPAR receptor, as well as some colon cancer.

Diabetes

Endocannabinoids intersect with diabetes on two fronts: food intake and PPAR (discussed previously). Appetite stimulation through cannabinoid actions at central CB1 can lead to increased food intake, but peripheral CB1 modulation has shown to increase fatty acid metabolism as well as decrease food intake (O'Keefe 2014). Central CB1 antagonism can cause unpleasant psychiatric side effects as was the case with rimonabant, so a synthetic, peripherally-restricted CB1R anatagonist that did not cross the blood brain barrier would lack effects on mood while preserving effects on peripheral fat metabolism.

Influence from dietary omega fatty acids and their effects upon fatty acid metabolism, are at play as well, which in turn affects PPARl. One hypothesis is that a high omega 6:3 ratio causes overactive endocannabinoid activity, which then can dispose to obesity (Murru 2013).

The size of the antihyperglycemic and antiobesity market will likely keep pharmaceutical companies working toward answers around the obesity/cannabinoid interplay.

Osteoporosis

Osteoporosis is most common form of degenerative bone disease and affects over 50 million Americans. Natural bone remodeling is affected by a number of factors, but usually begins to favor resorption with decreased hormone levels and aging.

Nonspecific CB1 and CB2 agonists such as anandamide and THC appear to tip the bone remodeling balance in favor of resorption, resulting in decreased bone mass. CBD inhibits GPR55, which in mice has been shown to inhibit osteoclast activity without affecting osteoblasts, suggesting that it could be valuable for osteoporosis prevention (Idris 2012). Genetically CB2-deficient mice develop osteoporosis-like bone structure , and selective CB2 activation with a synthetic agonist prevented oophorectomy-induced bone loss (Ofek 2006).

Following initial studies with CBD, other cannabinoids are also being evaluated for osteoporosis prevention, particularly those that are active at CB2 but lack significant CB1-mediated psychoactivity, such as THCV (R. Pertwee 2008).

Mental Health
One-third of pts with schizophrenia do not achieve adequate results with conventional treatment, despite suffering multiple side effects. Earlier studies indicating that cannabis could trigger psychotic breaks earlier in life did not specify CBD or THC content, but given the timeframe of the studies, likely there was no significant CBD component.

CBD has been shown to have much the opposite effect—calming the psyche. Effects at 5-HT have been recently demonstrated, which mediate a calming, antidepressant effect. Endogenous AEA appears to play a part in schizophrenia, since levels of AEA appear to correlate with symptoms in some patients. Following up on earlier case reports, a recent clinical trial in Germany showed that CBD and the associated rise in AEA had therapeutic effect in patients comparable to a conventional antipsychotic, but with fewer side effects (Leweke 2012).

Other Neurodegenerative Diseases

Parkinson's disease (PD)

PD is a neurodegenerative disorder characterized by a dramatic loss of dopaminergic neurons in the substantia nigra (SN). Several pathologic mechanisms have been proposed, including excitotoxicity and oxidative stress. In recent years, the involvement of neuroinflammatory processes in nigral degeneration has gained increasing attention. Not only have activated microglia and increased levels of inflammatory mediators been detected in the striatum of PD patients, but a large body of animal studies points to a contributory role of inflammation in dopaminergic cell loss.

Huntington's Disease

Known for its hypertonic chorea, Huntington's disease is neurologic condition with little treatment in conventional medicine. In postmortem brain samples, CB1 receptors are lost in the basal ganglia of Huntington's patients as well as mice, but the exact role in the endocannabinoid system in Huntington's is not yet clear. Through TRPV1 receptors, cannabinoids have potential to downregulate hyperkinesia, but only limited studies have taken place which indicated that Nabilone was not effective for chorea (al 1999).

Alzheimer's Disease

Deposition of beta-amyloid and subsequent microglial inflammation are hallmarks of Alzheimer's disease. In an animals injected with beta-amyloid, CBD treatment showed benefit in amyloid deposition and functional tests (Bachmeier 2013). Benefits in mouse cognitive functioning improved with administration of chronic CBD as well (Cheng 2014).

Dermatology

A number of the lesser-known cannabinoids as well as terpenes have antimicrobial, antifungal, and antiseborreic qualities. Topical cannabis preparations are safe and inexpensive compared to alternatives manufactured by prescription, and may offer a novel route to combat MRSA.

General References and Further Reading

O'Shaughnessy's: http://www.beyondthc.com/

Erowid: https://www.erowid.org/plants/cannabis/cannabis.shtml

UCSF Center for Medicinal Cannabis Research:
http://www.cmcr.ucsd.edu/

http://www.coloradodot.info/programs/alcohol-and-impaired-driving/law-enforcement/aride

Charlotte's web via Realm of Caring:
http://theroc.us/index.php?option=com_content&view=article&id=57&Itemid=388

High Times: http://www.hightimes.com

National Organization for the Reform of Marijuana Laws:
http://norml.org/about

Project CBD: www.projectCBD.org

National Highway Traffic Safety Administration:
http://www.nhtsa.gov/Driving+Safety

National Institute on Drug Abuse: www.drugabuse.gov/drugs-abuse/marijuana

State web sites:

AZ: http://www.azdhs.gov/medicalmarijuana/rules/

CA: www.cdph.ca.gov/programs/mmp

CO: https://www.colorado.gov/pacific/cdphe/medicalmarijuana

MN: http://www.health.state.mn.us/topics/cannabis/

NY: Bill No. A06357
http://assembly.state.ny.us/leg/?default_fld=&bn=A06357&Summar
y=Y&Text=Y

WA:
http://www.doh.wa.gov/YouandYourFamily/Marijuana/MedicalMari
juanaCannabis

Disclaimer

The information provided here is not intended to be a comprehensive review of the literature nor a substitute for medical education or legal advice. We believe that an understanding of the current state of medical research is essential to the proper preparation and dispensing of medical cannabis products. In this constantly evolving field, information can quickly become outdated. Website and other electronically-published information presented may be frequently updated and we recommend that the reader seek primary source information.

Photographs used herein are not restricted by outside copyright, obtained either by public domain or free stock photos.

Works Cited

1. AAO Complementary Therapy Task Force. "American Academy of Ophthalmology." *Marijuana in the Treatment of Glaucoma CTA - 2014.* June 2014. http://one.aao.org/complimentary-therapy-assessment/marijuana-in-treatment-of-glaucoma-cta--may-2003.

2. Abrams, DE. "Vaporization as a smokeless cannabis delivery system: a pilot study." *Clin Pharm* 82 (2007): 572-578.

3. Abrams, DI et al. "Cannabis in painful HIV-associated sensory neuropathy." *Neurology*, 2007: 515-521.

4. Adams, MD et al. "A cannabinoid with cardiovascular activity but no overt behavioral effects." *Experientia*, 1977: 1204-5.

5. al, Mueller-Vahl R et. "Nabilone Increases choreatic movements in Huntington's disease." *Mov Disord*, 1999: 1038-40.

6. Aldingtoon, S et al. "Cannabis use and risk of lung cancer: a case-control study." *European Respiratory Journal*, 2008: 280-286.

7. All Wales Medicines Strategy Group. "AWMSG Reference No. 644." August 2014. http://www.awmsg.org/awmsgonline/app/appraisalinfo/644 (accessed August 31, 2014).

8. Ambach, L et al. "Simultaneous quantification of delta-9-THC, THC-acid A, CBN and CBD in seized drugs using HPLC-DAD." *For Sci Intl*, 2014: 107-11.

9. American College of Physicians. *Supporting Research into the Therapeutic Role of Marijuana: Position Paper.* Philadelphia, PA: American College of Physicians, 2008.

10. American Medical Association. "Preliminary Proceedings of House of Delegates 2013 Interim Meeting." *American Medical Association.* 2013. 4-7.

11. —. "Report 3 of the Council on Science and Public Health (I-09) Use of Cannabis for Medicinal Purposes." *American Medical Association.* 2009. http://www.ama-assn.org/ama/pub/about-ama/our-people/ama-councils/council-science-public-health/reports/reports-topic.page.

12. Amtmann, D et al. "Survey of cannabis use in patients with amyotrophic lateral sclerosis." *Am J Hosp Palliat Care*, 2004: 95-104.

13. Andreasson, S et al. "Cannabis and Schizophrenia: A Longitudinal Study of Swedish Conscripts." *Lancet*, 1987: 1483-5.

14. Anthony, JC et al. "Comparative epidemiology of dependence on tobacoo, alcohol, controlled substances and inhabitants: basic findings from the National Comorbidity Study." *Clin Exp Psychopharmacol*, 1994: 244-68.

15. Bachhuber, MA et al. "Medical Cannabis Laws and Opioid Analgesic Overdose Mortality in the United States, 1999-2010." *JAMA*, 2014: doi:10.1001/jamainternmed.2014.4005.

16. Bachmeier, C et al. "Role of the cannabinoid system in the transit of beta-amyloid across the blood-brain barrier." *Molecular and Cellular Neuroscience*, 2013: 255-262.

17. Baker, D and Pryce, G. "The endocannabinoid system and multiple sclerosis." *Current Pharm Design*, 2008: 2326-2336.

18. Baker, D. "In silico patent searching reveals a new cannabinoid receptor." *Trends Pharmacol Sci* 1 (2006): 1-4.

19. Bayer Pharmaceuticals. "Sativex dosing." *Sativex.co.uk.* 2014. http://sativex.co.uk/healthcare-professionals/gps/dosing-titration-and-administration/dosing-and-titration/ (accessed 2014).

20. Bayer Pharmaceuticals. *Sativex Prescribing Information.* 2014.

21. Beal, JE et al. "Long-term efficacy and safety of dronabinol for acquired immunodeficiency syndrome-associated anorexia." *J Pain Symptom Manag* 36, no. 1 (1997): 7-14.

22. Behnke, M and Smith, VC. "Prenatal substance abuse: short- and long-term effects on the exposed fetus." *Pediatrics*, 2013: e1009-24.

23. Behnke, M et al. "Prenatal Substance Abuse: Short- and Long-term Effects on the Exposed Fetus." *Pediatrics*, 2013: e1009.

24. Berger, J and Moller, DE. "The Mechanisms of Action of PPARs." *Annu Rev Med*, 2002: 409-35.

25. Berger, WT et al. "Targeting Fatty Acid Binding Protein (FABP) Anandamide Transporters - A Novel Strategy for Development of Anti-Inflammatory and Anti-Nociceptive Drugs." *PLoS ONE* 7, no. 12 (2012): e50968.

26. Birch, EE et al. "A randomized controlled trial of early dietary supply of long-chain polyunsaturated fatty acids and mental development in term infants." *Developmental Medicine and Child Neurology* 42, no. 3 (2007): 174.

27. Bisogno, T et al. "Molecular targets for cannabidiol and its synthetic analogues: effect on vanilloid VR1 receptors and on teh cellular uptake and enzymatic hydrolysis of anandamid." *Br J Pharm* 134 (2001): 845-852.

28. Borelli, F. "Cannabidiol, a safe and non-psychotropic ingredient of the marijuana plant Cannabis sativa, is protective in a murine model of colitis." *J Mol Med*, 2009: 1111-21.

29. Brantl, SA. "Mechanism of platelet activation induced by endocannabinoids and blood and plasma." *Platelets* 25, no. 3 (2014): 151-161.

30. Brown, I, Cascio, MG, Whale, KW, Smoum, R, Mechoulam, R, Ross, RA, Pertwee, RG and Heys, SD. "Cannabinoid receptor-dependent and -independent anti-proliferative effects of omega-2 ethanolamides in androgen receptor-positive and -negative prostate cancer cell lines." *Carcinogenesis* 31, no. 9 (2010): 1584-91.

31. Budney, AJ et al. "Review of the validity and significance of cannabis withdrawal syndrome." *Am J Psychiatry*, 2004: 1967-77.

32. Carlini, EA, Mechoulam R, and Lander, N. "Anticonvulsant activity of four oxygenated cannabidiol derivatives." *Res Commun Pathol Pharmacol* 12, no. 1 (1975): 1-15.

33. Carter, GT et al. "Marijuana in the management of amyotrophic lateral sclrerosis." *Am J Hospice and Palliative Medicine*, 2001: 265-70.

34. Center for Behavioral Health Statistics and Quality. *National Survey on drug use and health.* Rockville, MD: Substance Abuse & Mental Health Services Administration, 2013.

35. Cheng, D et al. "Chronic cannabidiol treatment improves social and object recognition in double transgenic APPswe/PS1deltaE9 mice." *Psychopharmacology*, 2014: 3009-3017.

36. Clarke, RC and Watson, DP. "Cannabis and Natural Cannabis Medicines." In *Marijuana and the Cannabinoids*, by M, ed. ElSohly, 1-15. Totowa, NJ: Humana Press, 2007.

37. CNN. *CNN Health.* August 8, 2013. http://www.cnn.com/2013/08/08/health/gupta-changed-mind-marijuana/ (accessed August 2014).

38. Colorado Department of Transportation. *Marijuana and Driving.* March 2014, 2014. http://www.coloradodot.info/programs/alcohol-and-impaired-driving/druggeddriving/marijuana-and-driving (accessed September 20, 2014).

39. Colorado, People of the state of. "Section 16, Amendment to Article XVIII of the constitution of the state of Colorado." June 03, 2011. http://www.sos.state.co.us/pubs/elections/Initiatives/titleBoard/filings/2011-2012/30Final.pdf.

40. Curtis, A et al. "Cannabinoids for Tourette's Syndrome." *Cochrane Database of Systemic Reviews*, no. 4 (2009).

41. Davis, TC et al. "Literacy and Misunderstanding Prescription Drug Labels." *Annals of Internal Medicine*, 2006: 887-894.

42. DeLong, GT et al. "Pharmacological evaluation of the natural consituent of Cannabis sativa, cannabichromene and its modulation by delta(9)-tetrahydrocannabinol." *Drug Alcohol Depend*, 2010: 126-33.

43. di Tomaso, E. "Brain cannbinoids in chocolate." *Nature* 382 (1996): 677-8.

44. Dowd, Maureen. 06 03, 2014. http://www.nytimes.com/2014/06/04/opinion/dowd-dont-harsh-our-mellow-dude.html?_r=0.

45. Drug Enforcement Agency. "Controlled Substances: Adjustment to the Established 2014 Aggregate Production Quota for Marijuana." Notice, 2014.

46. Drummer, OH. "The involvement of drugs in drivers of motor vehicles killed in Australian road traffic crashes." *Accident Analysis and Prevention*, 2004: 239-248.

47. ElSohly, M. "Potency trends of Delta-9-THC and other cannabinoids in confiscated marijuana from 1980 to 1997." *J For Sci* 45 (2000): 24-30.

48. ElSohly, MA and Slade, D. "Chemical constituents of marijuana: THe complex mixture of natural cannabinoids." *Life Sci*, 2005: 539-548.

49. ElSohly, MA. *Potency Monitoring Program quarterly report No. 123 - reporting period: 09/16/13- 12/15/2013.* University of Mississippi, National Cener for Natural Products Research, 2014.

50. Englund, A et al. "Cannabidiol inhibits THC-elicited paranoid symptoms and hippocampal-dependent memory impairment." *J Psychopharmacol*, 2013: 19-27.

51. Espejo-Porras, F, J Fernanez-Ruiz, RG Pertwee, R Mechoulam, and C Garcia. "Motor effects of the non-psychotropic phytocannabiniod cannabidiol that are mediated by 5-HT1A receptors." *Neuropharmacology*, 2013: 155-163.

52. FDA. *FDA.gov.* Sep rev 2004. http://www.fda.gov/ohrms/dockets/dockets/05n0479/05N-0479-emc0004-04.pdf (accessed August 2014).

53. Flachenecker, P et al. "Long-term effectiveness and safety of nabiximols (tetrahydrocannabinol/cannabidiol oromucosal spray) in cinical practice." *Eur Neurol*, 2014: 95-102.

54. Furler, MD et al. "Medicinal and recreational marijuana use by patients infected with HIV." *AIDS Patient Care STDS* 18, no. 4 (2004): 215-28.

55. Gable, RS. "Comparison of acute lethal toxicity of commonly abused psychoactive substances." *Addiction* 99 (2004): 686-696.

56. Gertsch, J et al. "Beta-caryoophyllene is a dietary cannabinoid." *Proc Nat Acad Sci* 105, no. 26 (2008): 9099-9104.

57. Gertsch, J et al. "New Natural Noncannabinoid Ligands for Cannabinoid Type-2 (CB2) Receptors." *J of Receptors and Signal Transduction*, 2006: 709-727.

58. Gieringer, D et al. "Cannabis Vaporizer Combines Efficient Delivery of THC with Effective Suppression of Pyrolytic Compounds." *J Cannabis Ther* 4 (2004): 7-27.

59. Gonzalez, R. "Long-term effects of adolescent-onset and persistent use of cannabis." *Proc Natl Acad Sci USA* 40 (2012): 15970-1.

60. Gray, KA et all. "Prenatal marijuana exposure: Effect on child depressive symptoms at ten years of age." *Neurotoxicity and Teratology* 27 (2005): 439-448.

61. Grotenhermen, F. "Cannabinoids and the Endocannabinoid System." *Cannabinoids*, 2006: 10-14.

62. Grotenhermen, F. "Clinical Pharmakinetics of Cannabinoids." In *Handbook of Cannabis Therapeutics: From Bench to Bedside*, by E and Grotenhermen, F Russo, 69-116. Binghamton, NY: Haworth Press, 2006.

63. Grotenhermen, Franjo, ed. *Cannabis and Cannabinoids: Pharmacology, Toxicology, and Therapeutic Potential.* Binghamton, NNY: Haworth Integrative Healing Press, 2002.

64. Hall, W. *A comparative appraisal of the health and psychological consequences of alcohol, cannabis, nicotine, and opiate use.* New South Wales: National Drug and Alcohol Research Center, 1995.

65. Hall, W et al. "Cannabis use and psychotic disorders: an update." *Drug and Alcohol Review*, 2004: 433-443.

66. Hartmann, RL and Huestis, MA. "Cannabis Effects on Driving Skills." *Clinical Chemistry*, 2013: 478-492.

67. Hashibe, M et al. "Marijuana use and the risk of lung and upper aerodigestive tract cancers: results of a population-based case-control study." *Cancer Epidemiol Biomarkers Prev* 15, no. 10 (2006).

68. Health Canada. "Marihuana Medical Access Regulations - Daily Amount Fact Sheet." March 2007. http://www.hc-sc.gc.ca/dhp-mps/alt_formats/pdf/marihuana/med/daily-quotidienne-eng.pdf (accessed September 21, 2014).

69. Hogestatt, ED. "Conversion of Acetaminophen to the Bioactive N-Acylphenolamine AM404 via Fatty Acid Amide Hydrolase-dependent Arachidonic Acid Conjugation in the Nervous System." *J Biol Chem* 280, no. 36 (2005): 31405-31412.

70. Huestis, MA, Henningfiled JE and Cone, EJ. "Blood cannabinoids II. Models for the prediction of time of marijuana exposure from plasma concentrations of delta-9 THC and THCCOOH." *J Anal Toxicol*, 1992: 283-290.

71. Hwang J, Adamson C, Butler D et al. "Enhancement of endocannabinoid signaling by fatty acid amide hydrolase inhibition: A neuroprotective therapeutic modality." *Life Sci* 86 (2010): 615-623.

72. Iannotti, FA et al. "Nonpsychotropic plant cannabinoids, cannabidivarin (CBDV) and cannabidiol (CBD), activate and desensitize transient receptor potential vannalloid 1 (TRPV!) channels in vitro: Potential for the treatment of neuronal hyperexcitability." *ACS Chem Neurosci*, 2014.

73. Idris, AI. "The promise and dilemma of a cannabinoid therapy: lessons from animal studies of bone disease." *BoneKEy Reports*, 2012.

74. Jarvinen, T, Pate, DW, Laine K. "Cannabinoids in the treatment of glaucoma." *Pharmacology and Therapeutics* 95 (2002): 203-220.

75. Jatoi, A et al. "Dronabinol versus megestrol acetate versus combination therapy for cancer-associated anorexia: a North Central Cancer Treatment Group study." *J Clin Oncol*, 2002: 567-73.

76. Jiang, R. "Identification of cytochrome p450 enzymes responsible for metabolism of cannabidiol by human liver microsomes." *Life Sci* 89 (2011): 165-70.

77. Katz, DL et al. "Cocoa and chocolate in human health and disease." *Antiox Reox Signal* 15 (2011): 2779-2811.

78. Kay, GG, and Logan, BK. "Drugged Driving Expert Panel report: A consensus protocol." National Highway Traffic Safety Administration, Washington DC, 2011.

79. Kim, K et al. "AM1241, a cannabinoid CB2 receptor selective compound, delays disease progression in a mouse model of amyotrophic lateral sclerosis." *Eur J Pharmacol*, 2006: 100-5.

80. Kosel BW, Aweeka FT, Abrams DI et al. "The effects of cannabinoids on hte pharmacokinetics of indinavir and nelfinavir." *AIDS* 16 (2002): 543-550.

81. Kurtzke, JF. "Rating neurologic impairment in multiple sclerosis: an expanded disability status scale (EDSS)." *Neurology* 33 (1983): 1444.

82. Lamuela-Raventos, RM et al. "Review: Health Effects of Cocoa Flavonois." *Food Sci Technol Int*, 2005: 159-176.

83. Lazar, K and Murphey, Shelley. "DEA targets doctors linked to medical marijuana." *The Boston Globe*, June 06, 2014.

84. Leweke, FM et al. "Cannibidiol enhances anandamide signaling and alleviates psychotic symptoms of schizophrenia." *Transl Psychiatry*, 2012: e94.

85. Ligestri, A et al. "Antitumor actvity of plant cannabinoids with emphasis on the effect of cannabidiol on human breast carcinoma." *J Pharmacol and Exp Ther*, 2006: 1375-87.

86. Lutge EE, et al. "The medical use of cannabis for reducing morbidity and mortality in patients with HIV/AIDS (Review)." *Cochrane Database of Systematic Reviews*, no. CD005175 (2013).

87. MA Huestis, M ElSohly, W Nebro et. al. "estimating time of last oral ingestion of cannabis from plasma THC and THCCOOH concentrations." *Ther Drug Monit* 28, no. 4 (2006): 540-4.

88. Marcus A. Bachhuber, MD1,2,3, PhD3,4 Brendan Saloner, MD, MS5 Chinazo O. Cunningham, and PhD, MPP Colleen L. Barry. "Medical Cannabis Laws and Opioid Analgesic Overdose Mortality in the United States, 1999-2010." *JAMA*, 2014: doi:10.1001/jamainternmed.2014.4005.

89. Massa, F et al. "The endocannabinoid system in the physiology and pathophysiology of the gastrointestinal tract." *J Mol Med*, 2005: 944-54.

90. Matute, C et al. "The link between excitotoxic oligodendroglial death and demyelinating diseases." *Trends in NeuroSci*, 2001: 224-231.

91. Mayr WT, Pittock SJ, McClelland RL, Jorgensen NW, Noseworthy JH, Rodriguez M. "Incidence and prevalence of multiple sclerosis in Olmsted County, Minnesota, 1985-2000." n.d.

92. McPartland, JM and Russo, EB. "Cannabis and cannabis extracts: greater than the sum of their parts?" *J Cann Therap* 1 (2001): 103-132.

93. McPartland, JM et al. "Are cannabidiol and delta-9-tetrahydrocannabivarin negative modulators of the endocannabinoid system? A systemic review." *Br J Pharmacol*, 2014.

94. Medicine, Institute of. *Marijuana and Medicine: Assessing the Science Base.* Washington, DC: National Academy Press, 1999.

95. Mehmedic, Z et al. "Potency Trends of delta-9-THC and other cannabinoids in confiscated cannabis preparations from 1993 to 2008." *J Forensic Sci* 55, no. 5 (2010).

96. Mishima, K et al. "Cannabidiol Prevents Cerebral Infarction via a Serotonergic 5-hydroxytryptamine 1a receptor-dependent mechanism." *Stroke* 36 (2005): 1071-6.

97. Mueller-Vahl, KR et al. "Δ9-tetrahydrocannabinol (THC) is effective in the treatment of tics in Tourette syndrome: a 6-week randomized trial. ." *J Clin Psychiatry*, 2003: 459-465.

98. Murru, E et al. "Nutritional Properties of Dietary Omega-3-Enriched Phospholipids." *Biomed Res Int*, 2013.

99. Naftali, T. "Cannabis induces a clinical response in patients with Crohn's disease: a prospective placebo-controlled study." *Clin Gastroenterol and Hepatol*, 2013: 1276-80.

100. Naftali, T. "Treatment of Crohn's disease with cannabis: an observational study." *IMAJ*, 2011: 455-458.

101. National Eye Institute, National Institutes of Health. "NEI statement - The use of marijuana for glaucoma." Bethesda, 1997.

102. National Highway Traffic Safety Administration. "Drugs and Human Performance Fact Sheets: Cannabis/Marijuana." *National Highway Traffic Safety Administration.* n.d. http://www.nhtsa.gov/people/injury/research/job185drugs/cannabis.htm (accessed September 2014).

103. National Hospice and Palliative Care Organization. "NHPCO Facts and Figures: Hospice Care in America." October 2012. www.nhpco.org/research.

104. Natural Standard Research Collaboration. *Drugs and Supplements: Marijuana (Cannabis sativa).* 2014.

105. Niesink, RJ et al. "Does cannabidiol protect against adverse psyhological effects of THC?" *Frontiers in Psychiatry*, 2013: 1-8.

106. Nutt, D. "Development of a rational scale to assess the harm of drugs of potential misuse." *Lancet*, 2007: 1051.

107. O'Connell, FJ and Bou-Matar, CB. "Long term marijuana users seeking medical cannabis in California (2001-2007): demographics, social characteristics, patterns of cannabis and other drug use of 4117 applicants." *Harm Reduction Journal* 4, no. 16 (2007).

108. Ofek, O et al. "Peripheral cannabinoid receptor, CB2, regulates bone mass." *Proc Natl Acad Sci* 103, no. 3 (2006): 696-701.

109. O'Keefe, L et al. "The cannabinoid receptor 1 and its role in influencing peripheral metabolism." *Diabetes, Obesity and Metabolism*, 2014: 294-304.

110. Paul, BD and Jacobs A. "effects of oxidizing adulterants on detection of 11-nor-delta0-THC-9-carboxylic acid in urine." *J Anal Toxicol* 26 (2004): 460-463.

111. Pearce, DD et al. "Discriminating the Effects of Cannabis sativa and Cannabis indica: A web survey of Medical Cannabis Users." *J of Alternative and Complementary Medicine*, 2014: 1-5.

112. Pelayo-Teran, JM et al. "Gene-environment interactions underlying the effect of cannabis in first episode psychosis." *Curr Pharm Des*, 2012: 5024-35.

113.   Penumarti, A, and AA Abdel-Rahman. "The novel endocannabinoid receptor CPR18 is expressed in the rostral ventrolateral medulla and exerts tonic restraining influence on blood pressure." *J Pharmacol Exp Ther*, 2014: 29-38.

114.   Perry, Scott (Rep). "Congress.gov." July 29, 2014. https://beta.congress.gov/bill/113th-congress/house-bill/5226/text (accessed September 14, 2014).

115.   Pertwee, RG. "Pharmacology of cannabinoid CB1 and CB2 receptors." *Pharmacology and Therapeutics* 74, no. 2 (1997): 129-180.

116.   Pertwee, RG. "The diverse CB1 and CB2 receptor pharmacology of three plant cannabinoids: delta-9-tetrahydrocannabinol, cannabidiol and delta-9-tetrahydrocannabivariin." *Br J Pharmacol*, 2008: 199-215.

117.   Pertwee, RH. "The diverse CB1 and CB2 receptor pharmacology of three plant cannabinoids: delta-9-tetrahydrocannabinol, cannabidiol and delta-9-tetrahydrocannabivarin." *Br J Pharmacol*, 2008: 199-215.

118.   Petrocellis, L et al. "The endogenous cannabinoid anandamide inhibits human breast cancer cell proliferation." *PNAS*, 1998: 8375-80.

119.   Porcella, A et al. "The human eye expresses high levels of CB1 cannabinoid receptor mRNA and protein." *Eur J Neurosci* 12 (2000): 1123-1127.

120.   Porcella, A et all. "this synthetic cannabinoid WIN 55212-2 decreases the intraocular pressure in human glaucoma resistant to conventional therapies." *European Journal of neuroscience* 13 (2001): 409-412.

121.   Prentiss D, Power R, Balmas G, Tzuang G, Israelski DM. "Patterns of marijuana use among patients with HIV/AIDS followed in a public health care setting." *J Acquir Immune Defic Syndr* 35, no. 1 (2004): 38-45.

122.   Purohit, V et al. "Cannabinoid Receptor-2 and HIV-Associated Neurocognitive Disorders." *J Neuroimmune Pharmacol*, 2014: 447-453.

123.   Rappold, RS. "Legalize Medical Marijuana, Doctors Say in Survey." *WebMD*. April 2, 2014. http://www.webmd.com/news/breaking-news/marijuana-on-main-street/20140225/webmd-marijuana-survey-web (accessed September 20, 2014).

124.   Riedel, G et al. "Synthetic and plant-derived cannabinoid receptor antagonists show hypophagic properties in fasted and non-fasted mice." *Br J Pharmacol*, 2009: 1154-1166.

125.   Rizzo MA, Hadjimicaheal OC, Prreiningerova J et al. "Prevalence and treatment of spasticity reported by multiple sclerosis patients." *Mult Scler* 10, no. 5 (2004): 589-95.

126.   Rock, EM et al. "Cannabidiol, a non-psychotropic component of cannabis, attenuates vomiting and nausea-like behaviour via indirect agonism of 5-HT1a somatodendritic autoreceptors in the dorsal raphe nucleus." *Br J Pharmacol* 165 (2012): 2620-2634.

127.   Romano, B et al. "Inhibition of colon carcinogenesis by a standardized Cannabis sativa extract with a high content of cannabidiol." *Phytomedicine*, 2014: 631-9.

128.   Ruhaak, LR et al. "Evaluation of the Cyclooxygenase Inhibiting Effects of Six Major Cannabinoids Isolated from Cannabis Sativa." *Biol Pharm Bull*, 2011: 774-778.

129.   Russo, E. "Cannabis to migraine treatment: the once and future prescription? An historical and scientific review." *Pain*, 1998: 3-8.

130. Russo, E et al. "Chronic Cannabis Use in the Compassionate Investigational New Drug Program: An Examination of Benefits and Adverse Effects of Legal Clinical Cannabis." *J Cannabis Ther*, 2002: 9.

131. Russo, EB et al. "Agonist Properties of Cannabidiol at 5-HT1a Receptors." *Neurochemical Research*, 2005: 1037-1043.

132. Russo, EB. "Taming THC: potential cannabis synergy and phytocannabinoid-terpenoid entourage effects." *Br J Pharmacol*, 2011: 1344-1364.

133. Salim, K et al. "Pain measurements and side effect profile of the novel cannabinoid ajulemic acid." *Neuropharmacology*, 2005: 1164-1171.

134. Schubart, CD et al. "Cannabis with high cannabidiol content is associated with fewer psychotic experiences." *Schizophrenia Research*, 2011: 216-221.

135. Seely, KA, Patton AL Moran CL et al. "Forensic investigation of K2, Spice, and "bath salt" commercial preparations: A three-year study of the designer drug products containing synthetic cannabinoids, stimulants, and hallucinogenic compounds." *Forensic Science International* 233 (2013): 416-422.

136. Serpell, MG et al. "Sativex long-term use: an open-label trial in patients with spasticity due to multiple sclerosis." *J Neurol*, 2013: 285-295.

137. Sewell, RA. "The effect of cannabis compared to alcohol on driving." *Am J Addict*, 2009: 185-193.

138. Sharir, H and Abood ME. "Pharmacologic Characterization of GPR55, a Putuative Cannabinoid Receptor." *Pharmacol Ther*, 2010: 301-313.

139.   Sharir, H and Abood, ME. "Pharmacological Characterization of GPR55, a Putative Cannabinoid Receptor." *Pharmacol Ther*, 2010: 301-313.

140.   Sidney, S. "Marijuana Use in HIV-Positive and AIDS Patients: Results of an Anonymous Mail Survey." In *Cannabis Therapeutics in HIV/AIDS*, by E Russo, 35-41. New York: Haworth Press, 2001.

141.   Solinas, M et al. "Cannabidiol, a non-psychoactive cannabinoid compound, inhibits proliferation and invasion in U87-MG and T98G glioma cells through a multitarget effect." *PLOS ONE*, 2013: e76918.

142.   Srivastava, R. "Potassium channel KIR4.1 as an immune target in multiple sclerosis." *N Engl J Med* 367 (2012): 115.

143.   Su, D and Li, L. "Trends in the Use of complementary and Alternative Medicine in the United States: 2002-2007." *J of Health Care for the Poor and Underserved*, 2011: 296-310.

144.   Substance Abuse and Mental Health Services Administration. "SAMHSA.gov." *Division of Workplace Programs >>Drug Testing.* October 1, 2010. http://beta.samhsa.gov/sites/default/files/workplace/2010Guidel inesAnalytesCutoffs.pdf (accessed September 1, 2014).

145.   Sun, Yan and Bennett, Andy. "Cannabinoids: A New Group of Agonists of PPARs." *PPAR Research* 2007 (2007).

146.   The Criminal Law Reporter. *U.S. v. Randall, page 2300.* Arlington, VA: Bureau of National Affairs, 1976.

147.   Thomas, G, Kloner RA, and Rezkalla, S. "adverse cardiovascular, cerebrovascular, and peripheral vascular effects of marijuana inhalation: What cardiologists need to know." *J Am Cardiol* 113 (2014): 187-190.

148.   Thompson, D. "More People Choosing Hospice at Life's End." *US News & World Report.* January 2011.

149.   Tikun Olam. *Our Medical Cannabis Strains.* 2014. http://www.tikunolam.com/products.php (accessed 09 12, 2014).

150.   Tramer, MR et al. "Cannbinoids for control of chemotherapy induced nausea and vomiting: quantitative systemic review." *British Medical Journal*, 2001: 16-21.

151.   Tsai, J. "Immunoassays for the Detection of Cannabis Abuse." In *Forensic Science and Medicine: Marijuana and the Cannabinoids*, by M ElSohly, 145-178. Totowa, NJ: Humana Press, 2007.

152.   van der Meer, FJ et al. "Cannabis Use in Patients at Clinical Risk of Psychosis: Impact on Prodromal Symptoms and Transition to Psychosis." *Curr Pharm Design*, 2012: 5036-5044.

153.   Volkow, ND et al. "Adverse health effects of marijuana use." *NJEM*, 2014: 2219-27.

154.   Watanabe, K. "Cytochrome p450 enzymes involved in the metabolism of tetrahydrocannabinols and cannabidiol by human hepatic microsomes." *Life Sci* 80 (2007): 1415-9.

155.   Wolf, SA et al. "CNS immune surveillance and neuroinflammation: endocannabinoids keep control." *Curr Pharmacol Design*, 2008: 2266-78.

156.   Woolridge, E et al. "Cannabis Use in HIV for Pain and Other Medical Symptoms." *J of Pain and Symptom Management*, 2005: 358-367.

157.   Wu, Tzu-Chin et al. "Pulmonary Hazards of Smoking Marijuana as Compared with Tobacco." *N Engl J Med* 318 (1988): 347-51.

158.   Yazulla, S. "Endocannabinoids in the retina: from marijuana to neuroprotection." *Prog Retin Eye Res* 27, no. 5 (2008): 501-526.

159. Zajicek, J et al. "Effect of dronabinol on progression in progressive multiple sclerosis (CUPID): a randomised, placebo-controlled trial." *Lancet Neurol*, 2013: 857-65.

160. Zhao, P. "GPR55 and GPR35 and their relationship to cannabinoid and lysophospholid receptors." *Life Sciences* 92 (2013): 453-457.